Metabolic Confusion Diet

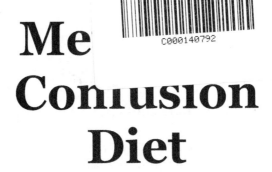

Beat Your Body at Its Own Game for Sustainable Weight Loss

Thomas Rohmer

Disclaimer:

This guide has been created for informational and reference purposes only. The author, publisher, and any other affiliated parties cannot be held in any way accountable for any personal injuries or damage allegedly resulting from the information contained herein, or from any misuse of such guidance. Although strict measures have been taken to provide accurate information, the parties involved with the creation and publication of this guide take no responsibility for any issues that may arise from alleged discrepancies contained herein. It is strongly recommended that you consult a physician, personal trainer, and nutritionist prior to commencing this or any other workout or diet plan.

This guide is not a substitute for professional personal guidance from a qualified medical professional. If you feel pain or discomfort at any point during exercises contained herein, cease the activity immediately and seek medical guidance.

Table of Contents

Introduction

Obesity. It's a problem in America that isn't getting any better. Companies spend millions upon billions to create addicting food products that set you up for failure.

Even if you have good intentions it's hard to overcome the vicious dieting trap where you lose weight only to gain it all back. Never once do you realize how your own body's hormones are fighting against you the entire time. With all of the odds stacked against you in your quest to be fit and healthy, it can seem like an impossible battle.

I know that's how I've felt. I've felt miserable thinking I had to eat healthy all of the time. That I had to eat small meals that left me feeling hungry.

Fortunately, it doesn't have to be that way. There is a way out and it doesn't suck. In fact, it's a good way to go about things.

What you're about to learn in this book is information that will change the way you view dieting. Gone are the days of fighting against your body. You'll learn how to eat your favorite foods and do so in a way that will allow you to continue making progress towards your goal.

Gone are the days of making yourself miserable only to slow your metabolism down to a screeching halt. You'll soon learn how to keep your metabolism churning along at a fast pace like a well oiled machine. And it all starts with the first step which is arming yourself with the right information. So let's get right down to business...

Chapter 1: Why Traditional Dieting Advice Has Failed You

You might be eager to jump right into the metabolic confusion gameplan, but there's some groundwork we need to cover first. It's important to understand why people end up in the situations they're in. There are a lot of factors that can lead to someone not being in shape like they want to be.

These reasons are especially true in America where close to 42% of the population is considered to be obese (1). Understand that some of these reasons will likely make you mad, and that's totally okay. It's important that you see the truth and realize that it's not your fault. You've been set up to fail from the jump. Here are some of the issues causing obesity:

Corporations

What do you think corporations care more about- their profits or your health? Take a quick look around you, and you'll get the answer quickly. There are fast food restaurants at every corner.

Turn on the TV and you're bound to see a fast food advertisement. Some fast food restaurants are literally open 24/7.

They make it convenient for someone to grab a bite to eat at 2 AM if they want.

Fast food restaurants are open on most holidays as well because they don't want to miss out on an extra day of profit. These companies literally pay their marketing team millions of dollars to create convincing ads to get you to try their food. Then their engineering team is creating ways to make their fries and burgers addicting so that you'll keep coming back for more.

It's a vicious cycle. It's not only fast food companies that are the problem. Think about soda.

Soda companies invest millions into advertising. They put millions into a team of engineers to help create the most addicting product they can. An average can of soda will contain around 40 grams of sugar.

Just stop and think about how much that is for a second. You would have to eat approximately 4 cups of carrots to match that! Even the majority of food products you see at the grocery store are tied to giant corporations looking to get their piece of the giant food industry pie. It's a competitive game.

What would you do if your livelihood was on the line? Would you want to give up your job or risk losing it? Would you just hope that you could find something better somewhere else?

Or would you do what you could to ensure profits stay high? I'm not saying this is an easy choice, but it's the reality for people who work for these large food companies. Essentially, these companies will pay people lots of money to work for them and help grow the company.

It's definitely enticing. Maybe these people don't understand the problem that they're helping to perpetuate. These companies take people's money and in exchange for that money they make people's lives worse with fattening foods that can lead to obesity and disease.

Don't get me wrong, I enjoy eating a fast food burger from time to time. There's definitely a smart way to go about eating junk food, but at a certain point, things went too far. It's a hard fight for most people to overcome simply because of the amount of money that's involved with trying to get you hooked.

Celebrities

Yes, celebrities have something to do with the obesity problem. We look up to celebrities as role models. We want to be like them.

We trust them even though we shouldn't trust every celebrity. This trust is where things can get dangerous for people.

If a celebrity recommends something that isn't healthy, you'll be more likely to consume that food because it's being promoted by someone you look up to.

Think of famous athletes who have an unhealthy meal. If you think about it, athletes need to fuel their bodies with good nutrition so they can perform their best. It doesn't make sense for them to eat a lot of junk food even though some athletes do!

Money speaks very loudly. Money can make athletes promote something that they wouldn't eat on a regular basis. The ironic thing is that this will help convince you to eat this food on a regular basis!

Whatever it is that a celebrity is promoting, you have to be skeptical of it. Yes, there is a chance that they used the product or ate that kind of food before they were paid to promote it. However, a lot of times celebrities will endorse a product simply because they were paid to do so, not because they actually believe in it. You should always do your own research instead of blindly going with the product or food item.

Your Environment

What kind of household did you grow up in? Were your parents super active? Did they cook or get take out a lot?

Chances are for a lot of us, our parents might not have been into exercise that much. They might've gotten fast food more often than they should have. When we're young kids, we don't think much of this behavior.

As a kid, eating junk food won't affect your energy as much as when you're an adult. Even as adults, we may not realize just how big of an effect the habits of our parents had on us. These bad habits of not exercising and cooking could be deeply ingrained in us by the time we move out.

This can be difficult to overcome, especially if you're not aware of it. You don't know any different than eating fast food because of how convenient it is so you continue to regularly consume it. It's not your parents fault, they did the best they could with what they had.

They likely weren't taught any healthy habits in school or from their parents so they simply didn't know. They were busy and didn't know what to eat or how to prepare healthy meals. It's not just your immediate family's habits that affect you. What about your cousins, aunts, uncles, friends and neighbors?

Education

Simply put, we don't learn about the best nutrition and exercise habits in school.

Kids in school today are barely given enough time in physical education class, and the type of teacher you're given can have a big impact on what you're taught. You could've grown up with a teacher who didn't care, just said "run laps" or just had you playing dodgeball the entire time.

I know for myself, personally, we would just play soccer everyday and play dodgeball on Fridays. I sure loved playing dodgeball on Fridays, but soccer I found to be a little boring. It's important to find ways to keep things fresh for the students so that they learn to fall in love with exercise.

Physical activity should not be viewed as something that is boring or something that feels like a chore. Being young is the perfect time to instill these habits, but unfortunately due to curriculum or maybe being dealt a poor teacher, sometimes school misses the mark. Also in high school, I never had to take a nutrition class to graduate.

I never learned much of anything about proper nutrition in high school. I then went to college and majored in Kinesiology, which is the study of human movement. As far as exercise is concerned, I did have to take 4 different physical activity classes.

These classes weren't anything too intense. It would be something such as a basketball class where you would show up and play basketball for an hour.

These classes were more so designed to ensure you were being active, rather than teaching you.

I also didn't have to take any nutrition classes in order to graduate. I say this to drive home the point as to how limited education can be in regards to exercise and nutrition. You really have to go out of your way and major in a specific type of health field in order to get the proper education needed.

This is simply not practical for everyone to do, and I don't see things changing to where a nutrition class and physical education class become a regular part of college's core curriculum. This really puts things on the individual to figure things out. For a lot of people, this unfortunately never happens, but you're taking the right step by reading this book.

Busy Lives

Simply put, we are busy. If we had an unlimited amount of time to exercise and meal prep, then I'm sure the overall health of people would be much better. Typically, we are rushed with everything we do.

You are rushed to get the kids to school and then to get to work. Then by the time you get home, you're exhausted and now you have to think about what to feed everyone after a long day. Or maybe you're going to school and working a job as well.

No matter what your scenario is, I can bet that it involves being busy. This certainly doesn't make things any easier, so we have to be strategic with the free time we do have in order to make the most of our health and fitness.

Lots of Bad Information

We live in the digital age. More information is at our fingertips than ever before. However, the obesity problem in America hasn't been fixed, and things aren't trending in the right direction.

This is surprising considering it's not hard to find plenty of information about health and fitness on the internet. The reality is that just because there's plenty of resources doesn't mean that the resources are sound. There's a lot of information out there that simply holds people back.

It's not because the people producing this information have the wrong intention. Sometimes the information could simply be too hard to execute over a long period of time. For instance, imagine me telling you that it would be beneficial to go on a two week long juice cleanse.

Sure, this could have some good health benefits for you, but is it really practical to be able to do that? No matter how well intentioned my advice is, most people would not be able to go three days on juices let alone two weeks.

However, if you take my advice and try out this cleanse only to quit, then you feel like a failure.

Then all of the doubt starts to creep in and make you wonder if you'll ever achieve your health and fitness goals. Another example of a myth being perpetuated is eating healthy to lose weight. It's been ingrained in us that in order to lose weight, we must eat healthy.

So we eat healthy until a scenario like a birthday party or a coworker bringing doughnuts to work comes up. We cave and eat something we "shouldn't have" and then feel guilty because the diet is "ruined." The truth is that you can definitely eat junk food in order to get in shape.

In fact, as you'll come to learn, eating healthy 100% of the time can indirectly lead to your metabolism backfiring on you. You can keep your metabolism firing off at a smooth pace by incorporating some of your favorite foods into your diet plan. This way you get the best of both worlds, but unfortunately this kind of information isn't known about and therefore isn't taught much! Luckily for you, you will have the correct information in your hands to be able to outsmart your body and get in shape.

The sad thing is that I don't see any of these problems getting better any time soon. There's more and more money that will continue to be poured into these different avenues.

This money will allow companies to continue to feed people the wrong information.

However, change starts with correct knowledge. Even once you have the right information in your hands, that alone is not enough. You must be able to execute on what you've learned.

You can't do that if you don't have the right mindset. If your past failures and limiting beliefs are holding you back, you won't be successful regardless of what you know. This is why it's important that we tackle your mindset before anything else.

Chapter 2: Your Past Failures Have Made You Doubt

I know you might be eager to jump right into the Metabolic Confusion Diet plan, but this is actually where most people go wrong. You must set the proper foundation for yourself before moving into the actual nutrition information. Imagine if you have negative experiences from your past or childhood that could still be affecting you to this very day. It simply won't matter if you know what to do; one way or another, your past will hold you back from achieving your goals.

What an Elephant and Running a Mile in Under 4-Minutes Have to Do With You Getting in Shape

When elephants are babies in the circus, the workers will actually tether one of its legs with a small rope. The rope is nothing amazing by any means, but the elephant can try as hard as it wants and it won't be able to break free. The crazy thing is that they will then do the same thing to tether an adult elephant.

They'll put a rope around one of its legs. The adult elephant could easily break free. However, the adult elephant won't even attempt to break free.

The reason for this is because it would try so hard when it was young with no success that it figures there's no point in trying now. The elephant thinks to itself, "I won't be able to break free." Clearly, an adult elephant would easily be able to break free from one measly rope tied around its leg, but it goes to show the power a belief can have.

An experiment done back in the 60s demonstrated this as well (2). A physiologist by the name of Martin Seligman would ring a bell and then give dogs that were part of the experiment a small shock. Through the powers of classic conditioning, the dogs would wince expecting a shock as soon as they heard the bell ring.

So far, there was nothing too crazy about this experiment and the dogs reacted the way you would expect them to based on the theory of conditioning. However, things got interesting when he would then put that dog into a crate with two panels. One panel would administer a small shock to the dog, and the other panel would not administer a shock.

There was a small barrier that the dog could easily see and jump over to divide the two panels. The dog would start on the side that would give a shock, and when that happened, the dog surprisingly wouldn't jump over to the other side. The dog would just lay down.

Seligman then experimented with dogs that he hadn't conditioned with a bell ring followed by a small shock. He would put these dogs into the crate and give them a small shock. These dogs would immediately jump over to the other side.

Yes, it is sad to think about dogs getting shocked, but this is how the theory of learned helplessness came about. Essentially, this theory states that our past experiences can teach us to not try to improve our current situation because we think doing so will be pointless. This is why the dogs would just lay down because they didn't think there was any point in jumping over the barrier.

From the outside looking in, that would seem like an obvious thing to at least try. This goes to show just how powerful learned helplessness can be. Of course, this doesn't just apply to animals, it applies to humans as well.

It was long believed by some that it was physically impossible for someone to be able to run a mile in under 4 minutes. This myth was absolutely shattered when Roger Bannister became the first man to ever run a mile in under 4 minutes. Since this happened, over 1,000 athletes have broken the 4-minute mile marker (3).

Some of these people have even been high schoolers! This reveals how powerful your beliefs can be when it comes to trying to achieve a goal.

How This Applies to Your Fitness Journey

The theory of learned helplessness is very prevalent when it comes to getting in shape. Maybe you've tried to get in shape in the past. You've tried multiple different diets and supplements to get more fit.

If they've all failed you, it can be easy to give up and not even try again. You might think there's no point in trying because whatever you try this time simply won't work. Of course, it's understandable to feel this way because most diets aren't that good and will cause you to fail simply by the nature of what you're expected to do.

At a certain point, most people say, "forget this; I'm going to eat how I want and at least enjoy it." This phrase or phrases similar to it are the equivalent to the dog just laying down and taking the shock instead of jumping to the other side. Instead of giving up for good, you need to stop and think about why you feel things are hopeless.

Is there truly no way for you to get in shape? Or is there no way you can get in shape and still have a balance with what you eat? Consider what you've tried in the past, and ask yourself if that plan was really the best to begin with?

Maybe your lack of success had less to do with your will or execution and more to do with the diet being bad. Or maybe the nutrition was sound, but you didn't take it that seriously. Either way, you must be honest with yourself and try to see what the root cause of the failure was.

This way you can move forward. If you simply just say, "this is pointless" then you could miss an obvious solution that's right in front of your face, much like how the dog could hop over a short barrier to escape pain. Taking a critical look at your past attempts to get in shape will keep your mind open and honest.

When we shut down and give up, so do our brains. Our brains want to conserve energy, and thinking can be hard sometimes. If you give your brain the opportunity to shut off and not have to think about a way to solve a problem, it will definitely do so. This will ultimately keep you stuck in your current situation.

A Few Examples of This in My Own Life

When I was a child, around 10 years old, I would regularly see commercials promoting fragrance spray for men. The commercials consisted of these shirtless models playing a sport of some kind like soccer, and women would be oohing and aahing over them.

I remember looking at the chiseled abs on the models and thinking to myself, "Wow they were really lucky to be born with a body that looks like that; I'll never have a body like they do."

Back then, I obviously didn't know what I know now, which is that you have influence and control over how your body looks. If you don't have visible abs, you can make your abs show via proper diet and exercise to get rid of the excess fat that's covering your abs. Sure, some people are born with better genetics than others, but at the end of the day, these models weren't born with a beautiful set of six pack abs, they had to earn it one way or another.

Of course, being a kid at the time, I didn't think to question this belief. I didn't ask myself a simple question such as, "Could achieving a body like these models even *be* possible?" Or said in another way, "How could I get a body like the models in this commercial?"

Instead, my mind was totally shut off to the idea of getting a body like the guys in that commercial. It just wasn't in the cards for me. This could be explained due to ignorance because I was so young at the time, but how many times does something like this happen to adults? Big or small, how often do we write something off or ignore something based on beliefs that aren't true?

Imagine if I told you that the sun revolves around the earth. You'd probably laugh at me and think that I was crazy! However, if I told you this same information back in the 1400s before it was first theorized that the earth revolves around the sun (4), you'd likely agree with me!

In the second scenario, we don't think anything is out of the ordinary because our whole lives we were taught that the sun revolves around the earth. In reality, we would both be wrong. We would be no different than the dogs getting shocked and just thinking this is how things are.

It doesn't hurt to question conventional wisdom to verify that it is correct. In fact, that's what this book is all about because the typical dieting advice doesn't work for most people. That's clear to see!

When You Question Things and Believe Wholeheartedly in What You're Doing

Growing up, I loved the game of basketball. I would always watch it on TV and play basketball video games. So naturally, I played the sport myself.

What's the one thing every basketball player wants to be able to do? Dunk! I couldn't dunk naturally, I had to improve my vertical jump in order to be able to achieve this goal.

So I would train using vertical jump programs in order to increase my vertical jump. I tried out three different programs and none of them did much for me, unfortunately. Imagine trying three different diets and failing to lose any weight.

How would you feel after that? Probably pretty defeated. You would question if this is meant to be or if you're stuck forever at your current bodyweight.

These are the types of thoughts that I was having. I wondered if I would ever be able to dunk a basketball. The thing was that time was running out for me.

I was a junior in high school and all of these programs had failed me up to this point. If I didn't figure something out before my senior season of basketball, I would never get the chance to showcase my new ability. Then I tried out my fourth vertical jump program.

This program was far different and unique from the first three programs I had tried before. It had unique plyometric exercises that I had never heard of before. Sure, the program was unique to me, but that didn't guarantee that it would be good.

However, for some reason that I don't fully understand, I had complete faith in this program. The program claimed that you could add 1" to your vertical jump per week, and I fully believed in that. Due to this belief, I was super eager to get started because I knew that this would work out for me 100%.

At the time when I bought the program, I was still in school. It was March, and I wouldn't be able to start the program until summertime when I wouldn't be participating in my school's regular athletics program. So for the next couple of months, I devoured that program.

I studied it inside and out. I read over it multiple times. I got all of the equipment the program asked for. All that was left was for me to execute when the time came.

When summer finally did roll around, I got to work and did everything that I was supposed to do down to the T. And sure enough, six weeks later, I was able to add 6 inches to my vertical jump. Now I was consistently dunking like nobody's business.

It all started because of the way I approached the program mentally. It would have been understandable to give up after failing three times in a row.

It would have been reasonable to go through the motions and give a half-hearted attempt at the program because I didn't fully believe that it was possible for me to increase my vertical jump. These beliefs simply would have held me back from achieving the success that I ultimately did.

How Are You Going to Approach This Book?

When it comes to the information in this book, you can approach things in a similar manner to the way I did with my vertical jump program. First and foremost, I want you to truly believe that the information in this book will be different from what you've known in the past. I want you to believe that this book is the missing link you've needed to be successful.

Quite a few people who buy a book never get around to actually reading it. Then there are people who will read a book, set it to the side, and forget about it. They don't take action on any of the information in the book.

This honestly isn't much better than not reading it in the first place. I want you to be different. I want you to read this book multiple times to really help absorb the information.

You'll pick up on things the second and third time that you didn't the first time. I want you to execute on the plan down to the T.

If you approach things with this type of mentality, you'll set yourself up for a much higher chance of success.

Overcoming Negative Conditioning

Now it can be easy for me to say, "Believe in yourself; believe that this time will be different." Unfortunately, things might not end up any different despite your best efforts. This could be due to deep-rooted beliefs or the way you view yourself.

The way you view yourself and how you think others view you makes up what is known as the self image. Ultimately, we act in accordance with how we view ourselves. Take for instance a car salesman who views himself as handsome and believes that he sells a good amount of cars because of his good looks.

If he wakes up one morning with a huge breakout on his face, what do you think would happen? His viewpoints of what he thinks other people think of him would change. The way he thinks about himself would change as well, and both of these factors would affect his performance at this job.

If deep down someone views themself as overweight, then they will act accordingly.

So for instance, if this person were to go on a diet in order to lose weight, things might start off good, but things will eventually get to a point where the person will engage in self-sabotaging behavior. They will start to ruin the progress they've made because being at a healthy weight isn't who they believe they are deep down.

Oftentimes, this will happen without the person even realizing it. This is why it's critical to improve the way we view ourselves and to overcome anything from our past that still may be holding us back in the present.

I'm Not Above This

Growing up, I was always very skinny. I would get made fun of with people saying things like I would blow away with the wind and that I needed to eat more. Some of it might have been light-hearted, but you never know how your words might affect someone else.

It was some of the things I went through in high school that drove me to want to improve my health and fitness. I wanted to build a chiseled and muscular body so people had nothing left to say about the way I looked. This is when I started to develop my love, passion, and even obsession at times with fitness.

I sold all of my video games so I could get enough money to buy fitness equipment. I turned my dad's tool shed into a gym. I was serious about this.

Being serious didn't mean I knew what I was doing though. I would eat six small meals per day. Each meal had to contain less than 10% of the total calories from fat.

I would also workout twice per day, once in the morning and once in the evening. Oh and of course, I would not eat anything deemed unhealthy or drink anything other than water! One day, I was working out in my dad's shed during a hot Texas summer day, and I nearly fainted from this excessively strict diet and intense workout regime.

It was at this time that I knew something had to change, and I had to figure out a better way to go about things. Through trial and error, I would find my footing and make it to where I am today. However, even to this day, even after all of the effort I've put into workouts and nutrition, I still sometimes see myself the way I did when I was in high school.

I'll look in the mirror and see my arms and think, "Dang it doesn't even look like I workout." It can be a pretty demoralizing feeling because it feels like a lot of wasted effort.

Don't get me wrong, I do receive compliments from time to time and that feels good, but I also still get comments about being skinny.

All it takes is one comment for me to get down on myself. For example, I was recently riding along in a two seater truck with two of my friends. My friend said I should sit in the middle because I was skinny.

I'm pretty good at hiding my emotions (just ask my wife), so I was able to go along with it. During the ride though, I was already planning out how much more dedicated I was going to be to my meal planning and workout efforts so that I could bulk up better. One comment like that can stick with me for weeks or even months.

I'm sure things might be similar in your life when someone says hurtful or triggering things to you. When someone says something hurtful to me, I usually get into my "I'll show you" or "I'll prove you wrong" type of mentality. However, other people may shut down or binge eat.

They can start to spiral out of control from there and eventually give up on their goals. All it takes is one comment, intentional or unintentional, to trigger old feelings from the past; this is where things can go downhill. We can also start to believe the lies that other people tell and accept them as truth.

For instance, if someone has a lot of different friends or family members telling him that he is "big-boned" and it's going to be really hard for him to lose weight, he might start to believe that it will be too hard and that it's not worth the effort. This is why it's important to have practices in place that you can use to snap yourself back into a positive frame of mind and smash through any beliefs that could be holding you back.

Exercise to Retain Your Frame of Thinking

If we want to stay positive when negative things happen to us or when negative things are said to us, we must recognize what is going on. Oftentimes, we're not aware of how we're reacting emotionally to a situation and therefore cannot change it. So first and foremost, get a pen and paper.

I want you to write down any past experiences or beliefs that have negatively influenced you when it comes to your health and fitness. It could be someone making fun of you, a rude comment a coworker said, someone telling you that your metabolism is too slow to get in shape, believing that you can't get in shape because you have bad genetics, or whatever else. Write down any experiences and beliefs you can think of.

Try to get to a total of at least 10 if you can. Then I want you to go through your list and rate each item on your list from a scale of 1 to 10. 1 meaning this doesn't affect you very much at all, and 10 being that this event or belief is extremely bothersome.

Then I want you to take the top 3 highest ranked items on your list. What you're going to do is reframe your line of thinking around those beliefs or events. You can do this for more than just 3 items on your list if you want, but 3 is a good place to start because these are going to be the things that have been holding you back the most.

For instance, let's say one of your beliefs is that you can't get in shape because you've been overweight for most of your adult life. We want to reframe that belief into something more positive such as, "There is no time like the present to get in shape thanks to my newfound knowledge." A statement such as this one is very profound because you're giving a reason why the statement is true.

Affirmations don't work well for some people and that's because your brain needs evidence as to why something is true. If you've been overweight most of your adult life and start to say, "I will get in great shape," your mind is going to look at all of the past years of failure and tell you that it's not going to happen because of x, y, and z.

After reading this book and getting the proper knowledge, you can move forward more confidently in a way that you never have before.

You can give your brain a legitimate reason as to why things are going to be much different this time. Said another way, imagine if you look at yourself in the mirror and say over and over again that you have six pack abs when you clearly don't. Deep down, you're never going to actually believe that and stimulate positive feelings from that statement.

However, if you were to say something along the lines of, "I'm capable of getting six pack abs because of my newfound efforts to nutrition and exercise," then you'll have more success. For a negative past experience, you could say something along the lines of, "I can overcome anything because of what I've been through." Or you could say, "hurt people hurt people."

This statement can help to remind you that oftentimes, it's less about what you've done and more so about an insecurity expressing itself in the other person. You don't have to write these statements down multiple times a day if you don't want to. I totally understand that's not for everyone.

Instead, write down your negative beliefs reframed into positive ones on sticky notes or on notecards.

You can place the sticky notes in places where you'll regularly see them such as your desk or refrigerator. If you write your new beliefs on notecards, you can simply read over them once in the morning and once at night.

This is how you'll keep those new statements at the forefront of your mind. It won't do you much good to reframe these beliefs and leave it at that. You'll soon forget about them and revert back into your old way of thinking. If we want to truly break through these beliefs, then we have to be reminded of them on a daily basis until it becomes second nature to us.

Overcoming Something That Happens in the Moment

The exercise I just shared with you is great for overcoming long standing beliefs that could be holding you back, but what do you do when something happens in the moment? What if someone says something to you or if you see or hear something that makes you doubt what you're doing? Negative thoughts that pop up throughout the day can set you off track.

It can sometimes take awhile to get back on top of things. Therefore, if you're able to stop negative thoughts in their tracks, then you'll have a much higher chance of staying in the state of positive momentum that's needed for you to see continued progress.

So what do you do when, in the moment, some event happens that triggers you?

How do you stop from getting down on yourself and having that potentially spiral out of control? The first thing you have to do is be aware of what is happening. Oftentimes, we're not able to control our emotions because we're not aware of what's going on with them.

Once you recognize what's going on, take a second to take in a deep breath and then count backwards from 10. This will give you time to process what just happened instead of instantly reacting to it. Then take the negative predominant thought you're having and reframe it in a positive way.

For example, my current goal right now is to add some more muscle to my arms. If I were to hear a story from someone else talking about how he has tried everything and it's been impossible to bulk up his arms, I would start to get discouraged and start to doubt. My mind would start to think things such as, "Will I ever be able to achieve this goal?" "Will my arms always be the size they are now?" "Should I just give up?"

A moment like this would be the perfect time for me to take a second to breathe, count backwards from 10, and then reframe the situation. In my case, I could tell myself something along the lines of, "Just because someone else has struggled doesn't mean that you'll struggle."

Sometimes the thoughts we deal with in our head are simply not true.

In this case, I would have no context as to why this other person is struggling to build muscular arms. Has this person truly tried everything? By "trying everything," has he given up on something after one day? How consistent is this person with their exercise and nutrition regime?

I have no context to any of this information and yet my mind wants to jump to conclusions based on a very limited amount of information. That's why this exercise is awesome to help bring you back to the present moment and keep your thoughts honest.

Setting Goals in a Way that Doesn't Make You Want to Fall Asleep

I'm sure you've heard about setting goals before; just about everyone has! Even with it being well known, hardly anybody does it (5). Studies show that people who set goals are more likely to achieve success than those without them.

When it comes to setting goals, you may just be thinking about it in terms of achieving financial success, but that's far from the case. You can set goals for other areas of your life such as relationships and especially for your health and fitness aspirations.

The question is though, how do we go about setting goals in a way that's actually effective?

Most people will set a goal and then soon forget about it. Honestly, I can't blame them. Setting goals in a way that's boring and unimaginative will certainly lead to someone pushing their goals to the side for something that's more exciting in the moment.

You have to set your goals in a way where you stay excited about them. This way you'll be motivated to work towards them.

Different Kinds of Goals

When it comes to setting goals, there are two different kinds: outcome and process goals. Outcome goals are usually what's thought of when it comes to setting goals. An outcome goal is simply the actual thing that you want to achieve.

For example, setting a goal to weigh 155 pounds would be an example of an outcome goal. On the other hand, there are also process goals. Process goals are very often forgotten about or even unheard of when it comes to setting goals.

However, they should not be swept to the side as they are critically important as well. Essentially, process goals are the steps you have to take in order to achieve your outcome goal.

Imagine for a second that you wanted to take a 5-day road trip.

Setting the outcome goal would be the equivalent to setting your final destination, which is definitely necessary! Imagine though if that's the only step you took and didn't plan out anything else. You would need to plan out which route to take, where to stop along the way, etc.

The details of the plan would be like setting your process goals. Basically, your process goals lead you to achieve your outcome goal. The process goals are the types of things you're going to be doing on a daily basis.

Far too often people just focus on their outcome goal. The problem with this is that any worthwhile outcome goal is not going to be simple enough to achieve overnight. It's going to take a while to achieve that goal.

When you don't see any immediate progress towards that goal, it can be easy to lose motivation and forget about your outcome goal all together. When you set process goals alongside your outcome, this problem is immediately eliminated. Process goals give you something that you can work towards daily to help keep you motivated and in a positive state of momentum.

A simple way to think about it is that your outcome goal is the final destination and your process goals are the roadmap to get you to your final destination. Now let's cover how to properly set outcome goals and process goals.

How to Set Outcome Goals Properly

When it comes to setting outcome goals, most people go about it incorrectly. There are a couple of key points that you want to make sure you're hitting on to get the most out of your outcome goals. The first question you might be wondering is how many outcome goals should I set?

I don't believe there's a good answer to this question. However, I've found it to be easy when I set one fitness related outcome at a time. This way I can focus all of my attention and efforts towards achieving that one outcome goal.

For instance, you might want to lose weight, but you also might want to tone up or add some muscle alongside losing the weight. Don't try to tackle both of those goals at the same time. What will likely happen is you'll end up achieving neither goal.

So instead pick one goal to focus on such as losing weight and once you achieve that goal then you can move onto the next thing. So now that you have an idea as to what direction you want to head in, what's the next step?

Simply stating that you want to lose weight isn't going to cut it, as you can probably imagine.

What you want to do is set a target. Put a number on how much you want to weigh. This will give your mind something tangible to work towards rather than saying something arbitrary and ambiguous such as, "I want to lose weight."

You could lose half a pound and technically achieve your goal. You might be wondering how you can determine your goal body weight if you're unsure of what you'd ideally like to weigh. What you want to do is simply take your best guess.

You're not going to know exactly what weight you're going to look your best at, so take an educated guess. Once you reach your target weight, if you determine that you still need to lose some more weight, you can always set a new target weight. I recommend setting a target weight as something that excites you but also doesn't feel unrealistic for you to obtain.

For instance, if an individual estimates that they need to lose 100 pounds, setting that as the goal might sound intimidating. Instead, the goal can be broken up into chunks. In this case, the person might set an initial outcome goal to lose 25 pounds.

25 pounds would be a solid step in the right direction, so it's exciting. But the goal isn't too large to where it feels impossible to achieve. Once this person loses 25 pounds, they can then set another goal to lose the next 25 pounds until the eventual 100 pound goal is reached.

Let's say a different person only needs to lose a total of 20 pounds. In this case, the person can set this as one outcome goal and work towards it until it's achieved. Finally, you want to make sure you attach a date to your goal.

This gives your mind a deadline that it needs to work towards and helps to create more urgency. You're not going to know an exact date to achieve your goal by, so take your best guess. If that date comes and goes, you can always set a new date.

When it comes to weight loss, setting a goal of losing 1-2 pounds per week is a good target to aim for. So if you were looking to lose 10 pounds, you could set your goal to be achieved 10-20 weeks out from today. So if we put this all together, here's what an outcome goal might look like for someone who wants to lose 20 pounds:

I lose 20 pounds of pure body fat by March 1, 2023.

The statement is also written in the present tense to help make things more real for your mind. The goal is also very detailed. Notice how I didn't simply say "lose 20 pounds." Losing 20 pounds could imply anything including water weight and muscle loss.

That would count as achieving the goal, but that isn't what's desired. What people really want when their goal is to lose weight is to burn body fat, so be sure to mention that if this is your goal. Now that outcome goals have been covered, let's dive into process goals.

How to Properly Set Process Goals

I've already covered why it makes sense to focus on one fitness outcome goal at a time, but what about process goals? Should you only have one process goal for each outcome goal? The answer to this would be no, definitely not!

You want to have more process goals than you do outcome goals. Each outcome goal should have a minimum of 3 process goals that go along with it. You could go up to 5 process goals or even more to attach to your one outcome goal.

This is because there are a lot of little things that go into achieving your fitness outcome goal. You're also not in direct control of what the scale is going to say when you step on it.

There are a bunch of little factors that can make a difference when you step on the scale such as how hydrated you are, did you just eat a meal, is it morning or evening, etc.

However, when it comes to your process goals, you do have more direct control over making sure these things get done. Completing your process goals on a daily basis will help to ensure that you're on the right track to achieving your outcome goal. The key is to determine which processes you want to focus on.

Which parts of the process of getting in shape do you tend to neglect? Do you not drink enough water? Do you not get enough sleep at night? Setting process goals to hone in on these types of things can help you stay on track. Here are a few examples:

- I drink half of my body weight in ounces per day.
- I get 8 hours of quality sleep each and every night.
- I prepare meals every Wednesday and Sunday.
- I exercise my body 4 times per week.
- I foam roll for 10 minutes every night before bed.

These are just a few ideas to help get your mind churning. Also there's no need to attach a date to your process goals because it's simply something that you're going to be doing every day or most days of the week depending on what the process goal is.

You could even take things one step further by attaching the word 'because' to the end of your outcome goal and then follow it up with your process goals:

I lose 20 pounds of pure body fat by March 1, 2023 because:

- I drink half of my body weight in ounces per day.
- I get 8 hours of quality sleep each and every night.
- I prepare meals every Wednesday and Sunday.
- I exercise my body 4 times per week.
- I foam roll for 10 minutes every night before bed.

Now you're giving your mind a reason as to why it should believe that your outcome goal is true.

How Often Should You Write Your Goals?

So how often should you write down your goals? Should you write down just your outcome goal? Or should you write down your process goals along with it?

Well for starters, as you can probably guess, writing down your outcome and process goals one time and setting them to the side is not going to be effective. What I recommend doing is writing your outcome goal and each one of your process goals down on notecards. Then review them first thing in the morning and before bed each night.

This way you're starting your day off with focus. You're keeping your mind focused on what you want to achieve. You can take things a step further by physically writing your goals morning and night.

However, if that takes up too much time for you then simply reviewing the notecards and keeping your goals top of mind will work great. You can also keep sticky notes with your goals on them around your house to give a constant reminder of your goals throughout the day. At the end of the day, there's no such thing as seeing your goals too much!

Chapter 3: Snooze Your Way to a Better Body

You might be wondering why I'm including a chapter about sleep in this book. Sleep can be another subject that at first glance appears to be unrelated to achieving your fitness goals, but that's far from the case. Think about it, the whole point of this diet plan is meant to optimize the way your metabolism and key fat burning hormones work.

As you'll soon find out, sleep plays a major factor in the way your body ultimately burns fat. It's something that isn't talked about nearly enough, and it's something that quite a few people need to improve upon. Let's go ahead and get you armed with the proper knowledge on sleep so that none of your other efforts are wasted.

How Sleep Affects Your Fat Burning Efforts

Sleep plays a major role in your ability to get in shape. We spend almost one third of our lives sleeping so it definitely matters. Most people don't have a good understanding as to how our hormones are affected by the quality of our sleep.

If these hormones are out of whack then we're just fighting an uphill battle that doesn't need to be fought.

Some key hormones that come into play when we're asleep are ghrelin, cortisol, melatonin, growth hormone, and leptin (6). Let's break down these hormones a bit further.

Ghrelin: this is one of your body's key hunger-control hormones along with leptin. When you're full, ghrelin levels decrease. They will later increase and signal to the body that you need to eat. Research shows that even just one night of poor sleep can lead to increased ghrelin levels and thus increased feelings of hunger (7). Imagine trying to fight against this all the time when it could be prevented by getting more sleep! It's obviously very hard to fight against your hunger hormones especially when you're tired. So it's understandable as to why people cave into these cravings.

Leptin: alongside ghrelin, this is your body's other main hormone to help regulate hunger. When you eat more and you're in a well-fed state, your fat mass will increase along with leptin. High amounts of leptin will signal to your body that you need to eat less so that fat burning can occur. When you eat less and burn fat, leptin levels decrease and this will signal to your body that you need to eat more. At first glance, leptin appears to be a very tricky hormone. As soon as you start losing weight, you're going to be fighting against your leptin levels. This is absolutely true if you don't know how to get around it, and it's a good reason why many people fail on their diet 2-4 weeks in. It gets to a point where people can't stand being hungry; that cheeseburger at the cookout looks really good so you cave in and eat something you feel like you shouldn't have. Not to worry though, I'll explain how to make the most of this hormone when I go over the metabolic confusion game plan. For now, I simply want you to have a good understanding of what the hormone does.

Growth Hormone: this is one of your body's key fat burning hormones. It helps with bone growth, muscle growth, and body composition among other things (8). The majority of growth hormone is secreted during the first phase of your sleep (9).

Cortisol: most people have negative associations with this hormone. It makes sense as to why because cortisol is our body's stress hormone. This is the hormone that elevates our body's flight or fight response. It increases our blood sugar levels and enhances glucose used by the brain to help provide more energy. Cortisol levels also increase in the morning to help us wake up. Cortisol may seem harmful, but it's very useful because it helps your body kick things into high gear. Imagine if you were in the woods and you came across a dangerous animal. Cortisol would limit other processes in your body that aren't essential in the moment, such as digesting food, and it would instead put all of the energy it can towards running away or fighting. There's no time to stand around and think; you need to make a move and make it quick. Cortisol helps you do that. The problem with cortisol is when we get stressed out in our day-to-day lives, and our bodies react as if we are running away from a dangerous animal. It's not good to be in a stressed out state on a regular basis. This is where things such as our digestion and our sleep can get disturbed. If cortisol remains high at night when it's time for bed then melatonin will be suppressed and that will affect sleep for the night.

Melatonin: you can think of melatonin as the opposite of cortisol, in a sense. Cortisol helps you get going in a hurry, while melatonin helps your body relax and fall asleep. Melatonin secretion is based on the time of day as it increases when it's dark outside. Blue light has been shown to decrease melatonin production at night. Blue light is a type of light that is produced by electronics such as a cell phone or TV. This is why I would recommend that you buy a pair of blue light blocking glasses or use an app on your phone that will automatically start blocking blue light at a certain time of the day. Taking melatonin as a supplement is a very popular thing to help people fall asleep at night. However, I believe in a lot of cases, this can act more as a mask to the problem rather than addressing the actual issue at hand. It can be things such as blue light or day-to-day stressors that cause melatonin production to decrease. The supplement can certainly help restore melatonin production to normal levels, but that doesn't mean there are no downsides. Your body can decrease its own natural production of melatonin if it becomes reliant on a supplement. This means that if you suddenly stopped taking the supplement, your body would have a hard time adapting because your melatonin production would be suppressed. You could slowly start to wean yourself off of the supplement for a smoother transition. However, in most cases, it would be better to address the root causes for lack of melatonin production in the first place, which I'll talk a bit more about later on.

Naturally, there are going to be exceptions to this. For instance, you might live in a place such as Alaska where during certain times of the year, it's only dark for 4 hours of the day. In a scenario such as this, your body is essentially going to be tricked into thinking you should still be awake. Melatonin could be one possible solution to combat against this.

Now that you have a better understanding of why sleep is so important for your hormones, you might be wondering what you can do to improve your sleep. First, let's go over why it's so hard for people to get enough sleep in the first place.

Why It's So Hard for People to Get Enough Sleep at Night

It's no surprise that most people do not get enough sleep when they go to bed. The CDC recommends that adults between the ages of 18-60 get at least 7 hours of sleep each and every night (10). However, a study by the CDC found that approximately one third of Americans aren't getting the recommended amount of sleep that they need to (11).

What's even more interesting is that Americans averaged 7.9 hours of sleep in the 1940s, but that has since decreased to 6.7-6.8 hours of sleep per night since the 1990s (12).

Unfortunately, I don't see this trend improving as time goes on. So why is it that people struggle to get enough sleep at night?

Why are these numbers trending in the wrong direction? Well, I don't think there's a clear cut answer to this problem. I think it's a combination of multiple different factors at play.

Different people live different lives so everyone's situation is unique. However, I do think there are common possibilities as to why sleep is such a big problem. The first thing would be the invention of electricity.

Many years ago, when the sun went down, there wasn't much of a way to have light other than using something like a lantern. Even then, there wouldn't be much to do, so you'd pretty much be going to bed when the sun went down. Nowadays, things are much different.

You can simply flip a lightswitch to keep your lights on and make it easier to stay awake. Not only that, but you also have modern age electronics such as smartphones and TVs that can take advantage of a wide range of streaming services. It's easier now than ever before to stay awake as late as you want.

You can stay up watching TV or scrolling on your phone, both of which constrain blue light that will stimulate you to stay awake even longer. I also believe that there are other factors at play, one being just the busyness of life. We have jobs, school, kids, unexpected events; there's just a lot going on, and sleep can easily get pushed to the side.

If you have a big project due soon at school or work, you might stay up late to finish it. It's not like you can sleep in to make up for going to bed late because you have to get up early to go to school or work. If you have children, anything that pops up in their lives needs to be taken care of regardless of whether or not it's your bedtime.

For some people, it's just not high on the list of priorities compared to other interests in their lives. For instance, my brother is a big basketball fan and enjoys watching the Lakers play. The only problem is he lives in a central time zone, and the games for the Lakers usually start late, sometimes at 10 PM pacific time.

This means the game won't even start until midnight for my brother, which means he likely won't go to bed until 2:30 AM. It doesn't matter if it's the weekend or a weekday, he watches every game. I'm not saying there's anything wrong with being a basketball fan as I certainly am as well, but I bring this example up to demonstrate how sleep can get pushed to the side at times.

Needless to say, we are busy people. So how can we improve not only the amount of time that we sleep but also improve the quality of our sleep?

How to Get More Sleep at Night

The first problem we need to tackle is getting more sleep at night. You can get a quality 5 hours of sleep at night, but that isn't going to do you much good because it's only 5 hours.

You need to have processes in place that can help you consistently reach the 7-9 hour mark if you're currently falling short of that marker. Here are a few ideas to help you out.

Set an Alarm at This Time of the Day

Everyone sets an alarm. It makes perfect sense as we need something to tell us when to wake up so we're not late for work or our other daily responsibilities. However, hardly anyone sets an alarm telling them to get ready for bed.
I know for myself, I can get so caught up in watching TV or being on my phone late at night that I start to lose track of time. Next thing you know, I'm getting to bed an hour later than I intended to because I was distracted. By setting an alarm at the end of the day, you can have something to alert you that it's time to start getting ready for bed.

For instance, let's say you want to go to bed at 9:30 PM. Set an alarm at 9:00 PM to tell you to start getting ready for bed. Now at this point, I recommend that you have a nighttime routine in place.

Make a routine that is predictable for your body in order to tell it to start winding down for the day. This can be something simple such as brushing your teeth, stretching or foam rolling, and taking a shower. Then once you're in bed, if you need something to unwind, you can read a book.

Reading a book before bed may sound boring compared to being on your phone, but it's going to be far better for you. The reason for this is because a book is less likely to send you down a rabbithole. You can more easily get lost in your phone.

Next thing you know, you're going to sleep way later than you originally wanted to even though you were already in bed. You also want to make sure you push up other routines or habits up to an earlier time of the day. People set the best of intentions to go to bed earlier but often fail because their routines stay put at the same time.

For instance, if your routine is eating dinner at 7 PM, prepping your lunch for the next day and then getting the kids ready for bed, you might not get to bed yourself until 10 PM every night.

If the goal is to be in bed by 9:30 PM but your evening routines stay put at the same time every day, then you're likely still going to stay on track to get to bed late.

Therefore, you should push up some of your evening routines to earlier in the day so you're finished with them at a time frame that aligns with your new sleep schedule. For example, you could eat dinner at 6:30 PM instead of 7 PM. This way you'll be in a better alignment to go to bed by 9:30 PM instead of 10 PM.

How to Improve Sleep Quality

Now let's talk about some ways that we can improve our sleep quality. Sleep quality and quantity go hand-in-hand. It does you no good to have one without the other.

So when it comes to sleep quality, the first thing you need to do is get your circadian rhythm in check. Your circadian rhythm is essentially your body's internal clock that tells it when to go to bed and when to wake up. The way that you can set a strong internal clock for your body is by going to bed and waking up at the same time every day.

This way your body knows exactly what to expect. It can start to release melatonin and cortisol at the exact right times.

If you're consistent with your sleep schedule, you may notice that you start to get sleepy at roughly the same time every night.

You might also notice that you naturally wake up early even on a weekend when you could sleep in. This is all thanks to your body's internal clock telling you when to go to bed and when to wake up. Things get messed up quickly when things are sporadic.

If you're going to bed at different times throughout the week, your body doesn't have a set pattern that it can adapt to. You might wake up one morning feeling super groggy even though you got 7-9 hours of sleep. The reason for this could be because your internal clock is off and you woke up at a time your body wasn't expecting.

Sleeping in on the Weekends

So what does this mean for sleeping in on the weekends? If you go to bed at 9:30 PM every night and wake up at 6:30 AM during weekdays then your body will have a consistent schedule to adapt to. However, when the weekend rolls around, if you sleep in, things will get thrown out of whack.

You could get plenty of sleep on the weekend and still wake up worse than if you would have woken up at 6:30 AM.

This is because your body is expecting to wake up at 6:30 AM, not 9 AM or something along those lines. I totally get it, sleeping in on the weekends is a completely normal thing for a lot of people to do.

However, if you want your sleep to be the best it can be, you need to keep things consistent for your body. Your body doesn't have a set internal clock for weekdays and one for the weekend. It doesn't know that your sleep schedule is 9:30 PM to 6:30 AM Monday through Friday and then midnight to 9 AM on Saturday and Sunday.

All it knows is that things have been consistent for the past 5 days and your body expects to continue on that trend. When you sleep in on the weekends, you're simply disrupting things. Now your body is thinking it needs to adapt to midnight and 9 AM, so when Monday rolls around, your body is confused again.

You might notice that it's harder to fall asleep on Sunday night and that you feel tired or groggy on Monday morning. It's going to take a couple of days for your body to get back into your weekday schedule, but by the time it does, it's already a few days until it's the weekend and you're on a different sleep schedule.

Hitting the Snooze Button

Another thing that is quite common among people is to hit the snooze button when their alarm goes off. The problem with hitting the snooze button is that it's not productive. This is simply interrupted sleep.

This interrupted sleep can possibly throw off your body's sleep cycle or circadian rhythm. This could make you wake up feeling worse than if you would have just woken up when your alarm initially went off in the first place. When you hit the snooze button, it's as if you're trying to delay starting your day.

This might be understandable if you're not excited for work or something like that, but snoozing is only going to give you less time to get ready in the mornings. You're more likely to be rushed, which will leave you less time to eat a proper breakfast, and you might have to stop at a fast food restaurant on your way to work to make up for lost time.

It can make your entire day feel like you're starting behind the eight ball, which can make it easier for you to fall for other temptations later on in the day such as a coworker asking you to eat out for lunch. You very well may have prepared your lunch for the day, but it won't do you much good if you left frantically out the door and forgot it!

If you're someone who regularly hits the snooze button, one solution would be to set your regular alarm for a later time. If you set an alarm for 6 AM but snooze until 6:30 AM, simply set your initial alarm for 6:30 AM.

Set Your Alarm Across the Room

The other tip I have for you to stop hitting the snooze button is to set your alarm across the room to where it's completely out of arm's reach. Taking this small action will force you to get out of bed to turn off your alarm, which in turn will make it much more likely that you'll stay up once you get up.

There's only one small problem with this advice...you think it probably won't work for you. The reason for this is because you likely use your phone as your alarm. How realistic is it for you to set your phone across the room?

If you're scrolling through your phone late at night, you're likely going to be too tired to get up and set it across the room. So what will instead happen is you'll put your phone on your nightstand as you fall asleep. Then when your alarm goes off in the morning, it'll easily be within arm's reach to hit the snooze button.

Yes, it's ideal that you don't scroll on your phone at all before bed. This would certainly make it easy to set your phone across the room before bed.

However, it's important to be realistic and understand that as simple as this tip is, not everyone is going to be able to follow it.

So what's the solution? Use something else as your alarm clock. It can be a separate electronic device or an actual alarm clock. Either way, you want to make sure this new alarm clock is set across the room.

Also make sure that you have the alarm preset for each day of the week. You don't want to set your alarm clock every night before you go to bed. This can cause you to sleep in because you're making the decision for when you should wake up in a moment when you're tired.

You could also not set an alarm, which might cause you to use your phone as an alarm and that may lead to snoozing. Ultimately, you can still achieve the benefit of this advice without having to give up scrolling on your phone late at night. Yes, it would be best to slowly get rid of that habit, but this is a good place to start nevertheless.

This tip will work for you if you try it out. I've been doing this for years, and it has allowed me to wake up consistently at the time I set my alarm. You just have to do it. Ask yourself what the priority is in your life.

Is it getting up on time and being disciplined, or do you secretly want to sleep in as late as possible? Be honest with yourself because there's not much required to execute this tip!

Sleep Debt

Hopefully you've found these tips on sleep helpful so far. I think it's also important to talk about what you should do on days when you are unable to get enough sleep. It would certainly be great if everyone could get the recommended 7-9 hours of sleep each and every night.

However, life does happen and sometimes we're going to fall short of that range. One thing that happens when you fall short on sleep is something known as sleep debt. Sleep debt is basically the difference between how much sleep you should be getting and how much sleep you're actually getting.

So for instance, let's say you normally sleep 8 hours per night, but one night you only get 5 hours of sleep. You now have a sleep debt of 3 hours. Then the following night, you only get 6 hours of sleep, and your sleep debt has now accumulated to 5 hours.

You can think of sleep debt similarly to having credit card debt. Credit card debt can add up quickly because of high interest rates.

Similarly with sleep, the negative effects of lack of sleep such as tiredness and lack of focus can compound if you continue to not get enough sleep (13).

So if you do find yourself falling short at times, what can you do? The first thing that comes to people's minds is sleeping in on the weekends. Unfortunately, there's no conclusive evidence to show this works.

There is research to show that sleeping in during the weekends won't help to correct metabolic dysfunction caused from lack of sleep (14). Another study followed 43,880 subjects over the span of 13 years and did not find a difference in mortality rate between individuals who slept less during the week and more on weekends opposed to people who got consistent sleep throughout the week (15).

If you do fall short during the week and want to experiment with sleeping in on the weekends, try it out and see how you feel. You may notice that it messes with your circadian rhythm too much and isn't worth it. The other thing you could try is taking a quick nap.

There is research to show that taking a short nap of 30 minutes or less can help to boost cognitive function and help to reduce tiredness (16). The last tip I have for you is a psychological one.

When you go to bed late and you know that you're not going to get a lot of sleep, what do you typically tell yourself?

Usually it's something along the lines of, "I'm going to be so tired tomorrow" or simply having a feeling of dread just imagining your alarm going off and wanting to sleep more. Now compare that to waking up on a morning that you're super excited for. Maybe it was celebrating a holiday as a kid or having a cool event that day.

You could barely sleep, and you probably weren't tired when you woke up. The point I'm trying to make here is that the story you tell yourself before you go to bed could make a difference. I've noticed this for myself, personally.

When I go to bed with dread telling myself I'm going to wake up tired, it inevitably happens. When I go to bed excited to wake up in the morning and tell myself I'm getting the exact amount of rest that I need (even if it's short of what I need), I find myself waking up with more energy. The way that I do this is by thinking of things I'm planning on doing the next day that make me excited.

I don't focus on thinking about tasks that I'm not looking forward to. This of course is my own personal experience, but it's worth giving a try in your own life.

Ultimately, sleep experts will agree that getting enough sleep each and every night on a consistent basis is what's best. Sometimes though, you do have to make the most of the situation you find yourself in.

Chapter 4: Metabolic Confusion Diet Game Plan

Now it's finally time to talk about the metabolic diet and how you can use it to outsmart your body to consistently drop body fat. Before I get into the actual plan though, it's important that you understand a few things first. I believe you should know the why behind the how.

If you only know the how, then you might doubt things if you don't see immediate results. Understanding the why will give you a solid foundation with your knowledge so that you can move forward with complete confidence.

Your Body and Weight Loss

How does the process of losing weight occur? To understand this, you must first understand that your body only cares about one thing- survival. It doesn't care if you have six pack abs.

It doesn't care if you hate the way you look in the mirror. It doesn't care if you think you're overweight. Your body will always do what it can to adapt to the situation it finds itself in to survive.

What's something your body needs in order to survive? Energy!

It takes energy for your body to maintain its normal daily functions such as breathing, digesting food, and organ function just to name a few. However, it's not realistic that you're going to be laying down and being still all day, and those are the only types of functions your body has to worry about.

You're also going to be doing other things such as moving around, and that's going to take quite a bit of energy as well. Thankfully, your body will be able to get the energy it needs in order to survive from the foods you eat. Food contains calories which is a measurement of energy.

The more calories a food item contains, the more energy it has. There's a baseline number of calories that your body needs every day just to maintain its daily processes. This is known as your resting metabolic rate.

When you consume less calories than your resting metabolic rate, what happens? Does your body shut down? No, of course not!

We would definitely not be here today if that were the case. It would be extremely tough to survive, and our bodies would not be good at their main job being survival. Your body will, of course, go somewhere else to get the remaining energy that it needs to function.

In this case, it will most likely go to your stored fat to make up for the difference. The stored fat is burned to be used for energy, and boom- this is how you lose weight! The reason I say it will most likely go to your fat stores is because in cases with very lean individuals, the body will tap into muscle to get the energy it needs.

This is not preferred by the body, and that's a good thing! This means if you have quite a bit of stored fat, muscle loss is not something that should be at the front of your mind. Conversely, what happens when you consume more energy than your body needs?

As you can probably guess, your body will store those extra calories as fat and save them for a rainy day. In the modern era, this may seem unnecessary if you have plenty of access to food. If your body does become in dire need of food, you can easily access it and consume it; so why the need to store the excess as unwanted body fat?

Unfortunately, we can't look at things from the modern age. We have to consider our ancient ancestors and even people in modern times who sadly don't have the same level of access to food that others do. Without this survival mechanism, the human species simply would not have made it.

Consider how our ancestors ate back in the day. They would hunt, and they would gather. They would move from place to place in search of food.

They wouldn't come across large animals all of the time. There would be times when food was scarce, and there would be times when food was more abundant. During times when food was more abundant, our ancestors could eat more.

The extra would get stored as fat and be there for times when food would be less available. This is what allowed them to survive. Things are much different in the present day.

We can drive to a grocery store and buy meat that has already been processed and conveniently packaged for us. There's not a way for us to change the way our body's biology works, so instead we must make the most of it. The way in which your body stores fat is really only half of the problem.

The other problem we have to understand is the fact that your body doesn't know when or where the next meal or source of energy is going to come from. It only knows things in terms of how much energy it's currently getting and how much energy it has in reserves, so to speak. So if you go on a diet to lose weight and eat low calories for a month straight, guess what that signals to your body?

"Oh no, I'm starving! I better slow things down to make the most of the calories I am getting."

Your body has no idea that at any minute you could splurge and consume massive amounts of calories if you wanted to. Everything is based on the survival mechanism.

This is how someone's metabolism becomes adapted to the lower calorie intake and ultimately slows down. This makes things tricky because now in order for you to continue losing weight, you must keep cutting your calories even lower. However, that will only make the process more challenging, and what's the reward for the extra effort?

You guessed it, your body's metabolism will adapt to the lower calorie amount and slow the metabolism even more. Again, this seems like we're having to fight against our bodies to make any sort of progress, but your body cares about living.

Lower calories for a prolonged period of time indicates food is scarce, and the body wants to do what it can to survive as long as possible. Back in the day, food being scarce was a regular thing, so it's a good thing that our metabolism can adapt and slow down so that we use less energy.

What This Looks Like in Real Life

Tell me if this story sounds familiar? Joey wants to lose weight. So Joey goes on a diet in order to lose weight.

He cuts out all junk food and eats nothing but healthy food. A week and a half in, Joey isn't doing too bad so far. It's been a little tough at times, but he's making it through. Now Joey is nervous because he has his cousin's bar-b-que coming up this week.

He knows there's going to be a lot of good food there, but he has to stay strong. He promised himself that this time would be different. He decides to prepare his own healthy meal at home and bring it to the bar-b-que to eat.

He knows people will look at him funny or ask him questions as to what he's doing, but he doesn't care. He's determined. He makes it through the bar-b-que without any binge eating disasters going down.

Fast forward two months later, and Joey is looking better. He's down 20 pounds now! People are complimenting him and asking him if he's lost weight.

It feels good, but deep down Joey is miserable. He feels like a rabbit most of the time, nibbling on some salad here and there. His energy is actually lower than it was before, and he always feels hungry.

Not in a starving way, but in a way to where he never feels quite satisfied.

He has also noticed that the weight on the scale isn't dropping as quickly as it was when he first started even though he's doing nothing differently. Joey isn't sure why this is the case, but he shrugs it off and treks forward.

Joey shows up to work just like any other day, but he actually forgot to bring his lunch in today. It's no big deal though because there's a healthy salad bar close by that he can stop by for lunch. Today is different though because his work catered lunch.

Street tacos are on the menu today, and at first Joey tells himself no way. However, after a few minutes of seeing everyone else indulge and being so starved of something like this for so long, he caves and decides to eat a couple of tacos. Now that the floodgates have been opened up, why not have some soda with it as well?

At the moment, it feels so good to eat some greasy tacos, but Joey feels guilty afterwards. He wonders why he ruined such a good thing that he had going. A couple of months have gone by now, and Joey has essentially returned to his previous eating habits, which consisted of sugary cereal for breakfast in the morning, vending machine snacks, and eating take out food 1-2 times per day.

However, after the dieting break, Joey's spirits are feeling back up; he decides to take another crack at this whole weight loss thing. This time he promises he'll be even more dedicated.

Maybe you can relate to our fictional character Joey here. Maybe you stay strong on a diet for months, then eat something you feel as if you shouldn't. From there, things either slowly start to fade or they go downhill in a hurry.

Maybe you're the person who can only last on a typical diet for a week and a half before you cave. Stories like the one above show how the dieting cycle can be vicious and how it continues on. Without a proper understanding of how to optimally burn fat, this cycle can happen to anyone.

A lot of people think that you just have to be more dedicated. If you're not able to eat healthy all of the time, then you won't be able to lose weight. So according to this belief, you essentially must choose between eating foods you enjoy or losing weight.

What a terrible choice to have to make. The truth is that you don't have to choose. There were things that were going on with Joey that he didn't even realize. It was just a matter of time before he ate something that he "shouldn't have." Let me explain further...

Our Good Friend Leptin

Remember the hunger-control hormone I talked about earlier called leptin? As a quick reminder, losing body fat causes leptin levels to decrease, which in turn signals to the body that you need to eat more and vice versa. Joey fell into the leptin trap without even realizing it.

He ate less calories by eliminating junk food from his diet. This caused him to lose body fat, which is a good thing, but his leptin levels continued to decrease. Unknowingly, Joey was fighting against his body's hunger hormones without even realizing it.

He thought he just needed to be more dedicated. That's why he felt guilty when he ate those street tacos. The truth is that this was inevitable.

Most people can only fight against their body's hormones for so long until they crack and can't take it any longer. This is why the majority of people who go on a diet eventually fail! It's not anyone's fault or lack of dedication. It simply comes down to the myth that you have to eat healthy 100% of the time in order to lose weight. That is false!

Metabolic Adaptation Otherwise Known as "Starvation Mode"

Something else you may have noticed in Joey's story is that his weight loss progression slowed down. He was losing weight at a faster rate in the beginning compared to the end before he caved. The reason for this is because his metabolism was adapting to the lower amount of calories he was eating on a daily basis.

The technical term for this is metabolic adaptation, but you may have heard of it referred to as starvation mode in the past. Your body isn't necessarily starving if your metabolism slows down, which is why metabolic adaptation is a more accurate term. If you've ever lost weight at a steady pace and then suddenly hit a plateau, this is why.

Either way, the point remains the same, how do you overcome things such as hunger hormones like leptin and metabolic adaptation?

How to Overcome the Trap

It's actually very interesting because the solution to this problem is often right in front of our faces. In Joey's case, the solution was right in front of his face being the street tacos. That's right, unhealthy food not only tasted great, but it's also a key component to aid in continued fat loss.

Let me explain. When you want to lose weight, you must eat less calories and/or burn more calories via exercise, there is no way around this.

Once you start losing weight, your metabolism will adapt and start to slow down.

Your leptin levels will decrease. This is normal and part of the process. However, at this point you have a decision to make.

You can continue to cut your calories even lower, which will work. You will continue to lose weight, however, your metabolism will continue to adapt by slowing down even more and your leptin levels will drop. The other decision you can make is to take a step back.

Strategically, eat more calories from foods you enjoy so that you can reset your metabolism and reset your leptin levels. Essentially, you're taking two steps forward and then taking one step back. This is far better than taking two steps forward and then exhausting yourself to continue taking giant leaps ahead.

In practical terms, you might lose 10 pounds and then gain 1-2 pounds in order to reset things so that you can continue moving forward. Overall, you're still down 8 pounds, which is what matters in the grand scheme of things. Later on, I'll show you exactly how to execute on this idea.

For now though, understand that eating foods like pasta, potato chips, pizza, hamburgers, brownies, and cake among others will help you get and stay in the best shape of your life.

These foods are high in calories, which will signal to your body that you're consuming plenty of food so your metabolism will start to restore itself. Eating a higher amount of calories will also help to replenish leptin levels, so you're not fighting against your body's hormones to burn fat.

This will help to reprime your body to burn fat. Not only that, but it gives you a small break and helps you to feel refreshed. Do you feel better when you work a month straight without a day off or do you feel more recharged coming back to work after a relaxing weekend? Things are no different with your body!

Putting Numbers to the Method

Having an understanding of how your body works is great, but now we need an actionable game plan that you can follow. How many calories should you eat per day? How often should you eat a higher amount of calories?

How many calories should you eat on days when you consume more calories? These are important questions to answer because if you're not sure then you could still spin your wheels, even though you theoretically know how to outsmart your body. So let's dive into those questions now.

How Large of a Deficit Should You Create?

As mentioned earlier, in order to lose weight, you must burn off more calories than you consume. In other words, you must be in a caloric deficit. There are 3,500 calories in one pound of fat (17). This means that if you want to burn one pound of fat, you must create a caloric deficit of 3,500 calories.

You could divide 3,500 by 7 days in the week to get 500 calories per day. This is a nice number for most people to aim to lose per week. An average daily deficit of 750 calories per day would equate to 1.5 pounds lost per week, and a deficit of 1,000 calories would turn into roughly 2 pounds of fat loss per week.

How do you decide what's best for you? As a general rule of thumb, the more weight you have to lose, the larger the deficit you can create. So for instance, if someone had 70 pounds to lose, it would be appropriate for that person to aim for 2 pounds lost per week on average.

If someone only has 5 to 10 pounds to lose, losing weight at a rate between 0.5 to 1 pound per week would be more appropriate. It may seem tempting to want to lose weight at a faster pace even if you don't have very many pounds to lose. The problem with this is you will simply get caught by the trap even faster.

Your leptin levels will drop quicker and your metabolism will adapt by slowing down at an increased rate as well. This is why crash diets don't work in the long run. It's better to be slow and steady. It will feel good to know that once you lose weight, the majority of it will never come back.

Calculating Your Daily Expenditure

Knowing how large of a deficit you should create does you no good if you don't know how many calories you're burning off in a given day. To figure this out, we first need to determine our resting metabolic rates, which we can determine by using the Harris and Benedict equation:

Women: 447.593 + (9.247 x weight in kg) + (3.098 x height in cm) - (4.330 x age)

Example for a 40 year old woman who weighs 70 kilograms and is 170 centimeters tall:

447.593 + (9.247 x 70) + (3.098 x 170) - (4.330 x 40)

447.593 + (647.29) + (526.66) - (173.2)= 1,448.34

Men: 88.362 + (13.97 x weight in kg) + (4.799 x height in cm) - (5.677 x age)

Example for a 40 year old man who weighs 90 kilograms and is 183 centimeters tall:

88.362 + (13.97 x 90) + (4.799 x 183) - (5.677 x 40)

88.362 + (1,257.3) + (878.217) - (227.08)= 1,996.799

Or

Women: 65.51 + (4.35 x weight in pounds) + (4.7 x height in inches) - (4.7 x age)

Example for a 40 year old woman who weighs 154 pounds and is 67 inches tall:

65.51 + (4.35 x 154) + (4.7 x 67) - (4.7 x 40)

65.51 + 669.9 + 314.9 - 188= 862.31

Men: 66.47 + (6.24 x weight in pounds) + (12.7 x height in inches) - (6.75 x age)

Example for a 40-year-old man who weighs 200 pounds and is 72 inches tall:

66.47 + (6.24 x 200) + (12.7 x 72) - (6.75 x 40)

66.47 + (1,248) + (914.4) - (270)= 1,958.87

Using this formula will give you the baseline number of calories that you'll burn off in a given day. However, this formula is used to determine your resting metabolic rate, which means you're primarily at rest for the day.

That's not the situation for most people. This is where it's handy to then multiply your resting metabolic rate by an activity multiplier. Here's a breakdown:

- Little to no exercise: 1.2
- Lightly active (exercising 1-3 times per week): 1.375
- Moderately active (exercising 3-5 times per week): 1.55
- Very Active (exercising 6-7 days per week): 1.725
- Extremely Active (physically demanding job or sports athlete exercising 6-7 days per week): 1.9

The thing with activity multipliers is you have to be honest with yourself. Oftentimes, we can put ourselves in a higher category than we actually are because we want to justify that we are more active. Doing this will only hurt you in the long run as it could cause you to not lose weight, and you'll be left wondering why.

This is why I recommend that you downgrade yourself one level from what you initially think you are. So for instance, if you believe that you are lightly active, then go ahead and place yourself in the little to no exercise category. It may not seem like a fun way to calculate things, but when it comes to calories you have to be careful not to overestimate how much you're eating.

Bumping yourself down a category will help give you leeway for potential miscalculations when determining how many calories you're eating. Let's continue on with our male example who determined that his resting metabolic rate is 1,959 calories per day and is in the little to no exercise category:

1,959 x 1.2= 2,350.8

This would mean that this person's maintenance calories are 2,350.8 per day. If this person eats right at 2,350 calories per day, he will not lose weight nor gain weight. If he eats more than this amount, he will start to gain weight. And if he eats less than this amount, he will start to lose weight.

From here, the next step is determining how fast you want to lose weight. For this example, the rate is going to be one pound per week. This means we're going to subtract 500 from the number calculated above:

2,351-500= 1,851

Therefore this person needs to eat 1,851 calories on a daily basis in order to lose one pound per week on average.

Once you determine how fast you want to lose weight, reference the following below to determine how much you should subtract from your maintenance calories:

0.5 pound per week: subtract 250 from your maintenance calories
1 pound per week: subtract 500 from your maintenance calories
1.5 pounds per week: subtract 750 from your maintenance calories
2 pounds per week: subtract 1,000 from your maintenance calories

Dodging the Inevitable

If this person eats 1,851 calories per day, he will lose weight. As time goes on, what will start to happen is his metabolism will start to slow down. It will go from 2,351 and slowly get closer to 1,851.

Your metabolism will not slow down to a point that is lower than the deficit you're creating. In this case, the metabolism will not slow down to a point below 1,851 calories per day so long as the person continues to eat that amount. Let's say the metabolism slows down to 2,000 calories per day.

Now the person is losing less than half a pound per week. Once the metabolism starts to slow down, most people will start to cut calories.

In this case, the person might cut down from 1,851 to 1,500.

Weight loss will then continue at the normal rate of 1 pound per week, but the problem is the metabolism will then start to slow down closer to the point of 1,500 calories per day. Obviously, this is a losing battle and it will make you want to quit. So how do we get around this?

You essentially want to take a break every 3-4 weeks. This means eating 1,851 calories per day for 3-4 weeks. Then the following week, you're going to take a break from dieting and eat maintenance calories or at a slight surplus for the whole week.

For example, after eating 1,851 calories for three weeks straight, this person would then eat 2,351 calories for the fourth week and continue that pattern. Or he could eat 1,851 calories for four weeks straight and in the fifth week, eat at a slight surplus of 250 calories per day totaling 2,601 calories per day. He would then repeat that cycle.

Doing this will help to keep the metabolism high and it will help to replenish leptin levels. Bear in mind, there isn't an exact science to this. You can tweak things as needed to best suit your lifestyle.

You might find that you can go a little longer before progress slows down. You may want to take a break slightly more often. Start by eating maintenance calories every 4th week or a surplus of 250 calories per day every 5th week, and see which style works better for you.

You may find that eating maintenance calories for half a week every other week is optimal for you. You won't know until you get started and try it out. Regardless, here are the main takeaways you need to follow to ensure your metabolism stays as optimal as possible:

-Take a break from dieting every so often (every 3-4 weeks is a good spot for most people)
-Don't try to lose weight too quickly (0.5-2 pounds per week is ideal for most people)
-Consume enough protein per day (more on this later)
-Incorporate resistance training as part of your exercise regime (also more on this later)

If you do these 4 things, your weight loss experience will be more enjoyable than the vast majority of dieters out there. You will also have a much higher chance at lasting success. Of course, there are still many questions to be answered such as how does exercise play into all of this?

Why does protein matter so much? How do I know how much I'm eating? And of course, what kinds of foods should I be eating?

This chapter was meant to give you a high level overview of how you can overcome some of the pitfalls that people commonly fall into. Now we're going to start to get into some more of the details to really help you fine tune things.

Chapter 5: What Should I Eat?

You now have a good understanding as to how much you should eat per day and how you can work around things such as metabolic adaptation and low leptin levels. Now, let's focus our attention on what kinds of foods you should be eating.

There are a ton of different styles of eating in existence today: low-carb, low-fat, liquid diet, paleo, mediterranean, vegan, vegetarian, and pescatarian, just to name a few. With so many options out there how do you know which one is best for you?

Realize This

Your goal is to consume a certain amount of calories per day based on calculations you can make from the previous chapter. Eating that amount of calories is what matters first and foremost. If you do that, you'll be heading in the right direction.

What you eat essentially determines how enjoyable or miserable you'll be when trying to eat a certain number of calories. For instance, if you go on a liquid diet or a low-carb diet, chances are good that you'll eventually grow sick of the diet.

There are so many good foods that are simply high in carbs that you theoretically would never be able to eat.

Same thing goes for the liquid diet. We definitely want to eat solid food that we can chew and enjoy the flavor. There's no point in eating in a way that you won't be able to maintain.

Even if you know how many calories per day you should be eating and that you need to take a break from dieting to reset your metabolism, it will ultimately do you no good. You'll eventually cave and eat something that you "shouldn't have." We hear low-carb diets being talked about all of the time.

We hear about all of the success stories. What we don't see is the aftermath. If someone lost 30 pounds on a low-carb diet, were they able to keep that weight off 6 months later?

What about a year later or 5 years down the road? On the other hand, eating nothing but junk food isn't a good idea either. These kinds of foods are high in calories and are mostly empty calories.

It's going to be hard to stay within your calorie budget. If you're not able to keep the weight off or lose it in the first place due to overindulging, then you're spinning your wheels. This is why I usually advise eating in a way that allows you to enjoy life.

You have to have a proper balance between healthy foods and unhealthy foods. The following is a good way to do that:

Be On Top of It 80% of the Time

When it comes to success with losing weight, most people have developed the mentality that they have to be perfect 100% of the time. This is so far from the truth! Imagine a baseball player, for instance.

If a baseball player bats .300, then this means the player gets a hit 30% of the time. If you're able to do that, you will have a long career as a baseball player because that's considered a very good batting average! No team is going to argue against a player batting .300.

In football, quarterbacks throw incomplete passes. Basketball players miss free throws all the time, and no one is allowed to guard them! If a basketball team averages making 80% of their free throw attempts, they will be at the top of the league, if not the top team in that category.

This means that they still miss 20% of their free throws, and that's all right! If professional athletes aren't perfect, then why do we think we need to be perfect when it comes to the way we eat? Treat it no differently than a basketball player and free throws. If you're good 80% of the time then there are no worries.

Just like if a basketball player makes 80% of his free throws, the coach will not be worried about it. This means that 80% of the time, you're eating healthy or clean foods. The other 20% of your calories can come from whatever you want.

You can calculate this into your daily calories to help give yourself a better estimation. Let's say you determine you need to eat 2,200 calories per day in order to lose weight:

2,200 x 0.8= 1,760
2,299 x 0.2= 440

This means that of your allotted 2,200 calories for the day, approximately 1,760 of them need to come from clean sources. 440 of them can come from whatever you want. Now on the 4th week, you decide to eat maintenance calories. In this case, that's 2,700 since you're losing weight at a rate of 1 pound per week:

2,700 x 0.8= 2,160
2,700 x 0.2= 540

The same premise applies here; eat roughly 2,160 of your total calories from clean sources and the remaining 540 from whatever you want. The cool thing is you don't have to think of this as strictly a daily thing. Maybe there's a nice restaurant where you want to eat, or you simply want to enjoy a fast food meal.

If you're only allowed 440 calories per day from junk food and you want to eat a fast food meal that's 900 calories, what do you do? Simply eat clean for an entire day (100% of your 2,200 calories for the day comes from clean sources) and now you can "rollover" those junk food calories into the next day. Now, instead of only being allowed 440 calories from unhealthy foods, 880 of your 2,200 calories for the day can come from junk food.

This would allow you to be able to eat the fast food meal guilt-free. Maybe you do enjoy small treats on a daily basis such as a bag of chips or a couple of cookies. Whatever the case is, bear in mind that this isn't something you need to be spot on with.

It's simply meant to give guidance on having balance in your nutrition plan. So why does eating healthy matter at all then? If you're able to control yourself and stay within a certain budget, what's the big deal?

Let's dive a bit deeper into the difference between healthy and unhealthy foods. Hopefully this will shed some light as to why striking a balance between the two is so important.

The Difference Between Healthy and Unhealthy Foods

Have you ever stopped and thought about what makes something healthy and what makes something else unhealthy? When we think of a red apple, everybody would think of that food item as healthy. When we think of pizza, we think of that food as unhealthy.

Why is that? What is it that makes an apple healthy and pizza unhealthy? I think if 20 different people were asked this question, you would certainly end up with a bunch of different answers.

This is for a good reason because ultimately, I do believe it's hard to pinpoint exactly what makes something healthy as opposed to unhealthy. However, there are some different factors we can look at that can help us get a good understanding where something lies on the healthy and unhealthy spectrum. One of the first things you could look at is the number of ingredients a food contains.
Oftentimes foods such as snack bars, pastries, deli meats, and cereals among plenty of others things will contain things such as preservatives, food dyes, or high fructose corn syrup. These ingredients are meant to help the food last longer, look a certain color, or help the food taste better. Research definitely shows that ingredients such as high fructose corn syrup are not that good for us (18).

Foods such as broccoli aren't going to contain ingredients such as xanthan gum, red 40, or anything of that nature, which is one sign you can look at as to why it's a healthier option. The second thing you can look at is nutrients. Let's take an orange, for example.

This hypothetical orange contains 80 calories and 15 grams of sugar. On the other hand, you could have 80 calories worth of a pastry that also contains a similar amount of sugar that the orange does. So if both food items contain 80 calories and a similar amount of sugar, what's the big deal?

The difference lies in the quality of those calories. The orange is going to provide you with a powerful punch of vitamin C along with some other nutrients such as vitamin A and calcium. Meanwhile, the pastry is going to provide you with mostly empty calories.

Empty calories are calories that provide you with little to no nutritional value. Empty calories are usually going to be things such as simple sugars or trans fat. Something such as a pastry is going to predominantly contain nothing but simple sugars, which means that the majority of your calories are going to be from sugar.

These calories won't do much to get you full or help you stay full. This means you'll have to eat more in order to feel satisfied.

This is a big problem if you're trying to limit your caloric intake in an effort to lose weight.

Imagine 100 calories worth of potato chips. That's barely going to be over half of an ounce. Now imagine 100 calories worth of kale.

That's going to be nearly 3 cups of kale to reach that amount! This goes to show you how quickly junk food calories can add up. You also get some wiggle room when you eat healthy.

It would be really hard to eat almost 3 cups of kale to reach 100 calories. This goes to show that it's hard to overeat nutrient dense foods. That's not the only problem you have to deal with when it comes to unhealthy foods.

A pastry is also going to rank very high on the glycemic index (GI) scale. The glycemic index is a ranking of how fast it takes certain foods to raise blood sugar levels. If a food item ranks high on the glycemic index scale, that means it will raise blood sugar levels very fast.

Conversely, if a food item has a very low ranking on the GI scale, this means it will take longer for that food item to raise your blood sugar levels. Something such as a pastry is going to have a very high ranking on the GI scale. Something such as spinach is going to have a very low ranking on the GI scale.

The problem with raising your blood sugar levels so quickly is that they will crash and leave you susceptible to swings in energy and hunger. Just imagine when you were a kid and maybe ate too much candy. You got a sugar rush and were full of energy, but soon enough you crashed and took a nap.

By consuming a diet centered more around low ranking GI food items, you can have a better control over your energy levels and you'll be less likely to find yourself hungry at random times of the day. You might be thinking it's so unfair that foods that taste good can really make it troublesome for us to get and stay in shape. It's totally reasonable to think that way.

However, it is for good reason that we are drawn to foods that are high in sugar and fat. It all comes back to our ancestors. Again, food back in the day was scarce.

So if you happened to come across some honey for example, it would be best to take full advantage of it. The simple sugars would provide our ancestors with a quick source of energy and calories. On the other hand, fat contains more calories per gram compared to protein or carbs.

Therefore, you essentially got more of a bang-for-your-buck, so to speak. Fast forward to the present day, and simple sugars and foods high in fat are all around us.

The extra calories from fat really aren't necessary in a lot of cases, and most situations don't call for quick sources of energy that simple sugars provide us with.

However, these kinds of foods are here to stay, so we might as well figure out a way to make the most of it. Rather than try to repress our instinctual desires towards these foods, we must strike a balance as mentioned earlier. After reading this section, you might not think there's much of a benefit to unhealthy foods, but that simply isn't the case as you're about to find out.

Why Unhealthy Foods Are Still Important

So what's the deal with unhealthy foods? How can they help us in our quest to reach and maintain our fitness goals? First and foremost, we are drawn to certain types of foods.

Naturally, the average person is going to think that ice cream tastes better than collard greens. Our ancestors needed these kinds of foods to help with survival and we still crave them to this day. So why should we try to run away from that completely?

We just have to be smart in how we go about it. Our ancestors didn't eat simple sugars all of the time because they didn't have access to it 24/7.

Present day, we do have access to simple sugars 24/7 so we just have to have some control over it.

In some cases, when you completely repress something out of your life, it just makes you want it that much more. In the case of food, if you really desire a juicy cheeseburger, but you constantly tell yourself no, eventually you're going to cave and get a cheeseburger with large fries, soda, and a milkshake. You're going to go all out!

Rather, it's better to tell yourself to wait until the weekend or to wait just a few days and then you can have the cheeseburger. Now you're eating something that you desire in a controlled manner to where it's not going to harm your progress. Secondly, eating food that's not the best for you gives you a break from the monotony and the grind, so to speak.

How do you feel when you work 7 days in a row? You probably feel pretty worn out and exhausted. Do you go into work on Monday feeling refreshed at all?

I'd imagine not! That's typically not the way things go though. Usually, the typical person will work 5 days in a row and then have 2 days of rest.

This way you can hopefully come back into work on Monday feeling refreshed. Eating healthy foods all of the time is no different than working 7 days a week.

What would eventually happen if you never took a day off in the workplace?

You would become burnt out, and your performance would start to suffer. You might get short with your coworkers. Things are literally no different with your diet.

Eating healthy 100% of the time for a month straight is the equivalent to working everyday for a month straight. Most people would not think that's a healthy work-life balance, and our nutrition plan needs to be viewed the same way. Thirdly, junk food helps you not look like a health nut.

I remember when I was first getting into health and fitness, I did not eat any junk food. One morning after cross country practice, my coach brought doughnuts. I refused to eat one.

My coach said, "One doughnut isn't going to cause you to gain fat. Your body needs some fat for survival." Looking back on this situation, my coach had the right idea.

One doughnut was not going to hurt me, especially considering I just ran multiple miles during practice! Additionally, on my 17th birthday, I had a party at my grandma's house to celebrate. I didn't eat any of my own birthday cake!

There's no telling how that made my mom feel. She really wanted me to eat a slice, but I simply wasn't having it. What did I really gain from not eating cake in that situation?

What did other people at the party think? There were plenty of times where my family would eat delicious bar-b-que or chocolate chip cookies, and I can remember just staring at the cookies wanting one so badly. I was good at resisting temptations.

Instead of getting bar-b-que with the rest of my family, I would instead eat some brown rice and tuna. Boring! For the typical person, there are going to be plenty of life events and things that come up on a semi-regular basis where you're going to be around unhealthy food.

Cookouts during the summer, weddings, work events, birthday parties, bachelor/bachelorette parties, you name it, it's going to be something you have to handle appropriately. Take it from me, it's not worth it. Think of all the amazing life events that you simply wouldn't get to enjoy to the fullest because you feel the need to be extreme with your diet plan.

Going to a party and having to bring your own meal prep container with brown rice and chicken simply isn't fun. I'm not the type of person who likes to draw attention to myself.

Bringing my own meal prep container is simply going to make me stand out in a way that will make me feel uncomfortable.

Plus everyone else will be eating delicious food and it will be hard to avoid temptation! I'm not going to look back on my life and be proud of the dedication I showed during parties. Instead, I look back on those moments in my life wishing I would've enjoyed them because it wouldn't have made a big difference in the long run.

Not only that, but eating junk food gives you a break from having to cook and clean up afterwards. Sometimes after an exhausting day, the last thing the average person wants to do is cook and then have a bunch of dishes to clean up afterwards. Finally, there's also research to show that not restricting yourself to healthy foods only leads to better diet adherence and is less likely to lead to eating disorders (19)(20).

The Importance of Protein

There are three macronutrients: protein, carbs, and fat. Each one has its own benefits that it brings to the table. Over the years, each macronutrient has had its share of being viewed under the microscope.

Low-fat diets and fat-free foods became quite popular during the 1980s and 90s, and they are still prevalent even today.

Part of the reasoning behind this methodology is the fact that fat contains over twice the amount of calories per gram compared to carbs or protein. Reducing fat intake would therefore help to reduce the overall amount of calories consumed, thus making it easier to create a caloric deficit needed for weight loss.

Interestingly enough, some reduced-fat or fat-free version of products still contain a similar amount of overall calories when compared to the original version. Therefore, you're not exactly cutting back by going fat-free. Additionally, not all fats are bad.

Fat is a good source of energy for your body and helps with cell function and regulation of body temperature. Just because fat contains more calories per gram doesn't mean that all fat or most of it needs to go. Yes, there are bad fats such as trans fat.

Most trans fats are artificially made in an effort to make certain food products last longer. Trans fats have been shown to increase bad cholesterol levels (LDL) and increase risk of cardiovascular disease (21). However, there are also good fats such as mono and polyunsaturated fats.

Unsaturated fats have been shown to decrease LDL levels and reduce risk for heart disease (22). Up next, we have carbs. Carbs are the macronutrient that are going through the wringer right now.

Carbs have recently developed a bad reputation because they can raise blood sugar levels and cause diabetes and heart disease (23).

However, all carbs should not be to blame for this. It's really the refined simple carbohydrates that are to blame for these issues. Complex carbs are foods such as brown rice, fruits, vegetables, and whole wheat bread.

Simple refined carbs undergo a process that strips the food of certain nutrients and fiber. Some examples of simple carbs would include soda, pastries, candy bars, white bread, white pastas, and white rice. Simple carbs are the type of carbohydrates you'll see that rank high on the GI scale, which is a bad thing for your blood sugar levels.

If you're constantly spiking your blood sugar levels, your pancreas must produce more insulin in order to keep up with the demands. Insulin is what allows your body to shuttle that sugar (glucose) into your body's cells. Over time with overconsumption of sugar, your body will start to become insulin resistant, and the pancreas will no longer be able to keep up with the demands being placed on it.

This is where people have to take insulin to help regulate the body's blood sugar levels and avoid hyperglycemia. The main function of carbohydrates is to be your body's first source of energy.

I believe that carbs should be a part of someone's nutrition plan, consisting primarily of complex, but also some simple carbs for enjoyment and long-term adherence.

Finally, we have protein, which is considered to be the golden child of the three macronutrients. Protein is everywhere you look now. Companies are all jumping on the high-protein craze making products that are high in protein from drinks to snack bars and more.

It wasn't always this way for protein though. Back in the early 1900s, some believed that the bacteria in protein could cause digestive issues and that carbs were the superior macronutrient (24). So yes, even protein has gone under some scrutiny back in the day.

It won't surprise me if people 100 years from now look back and wonder why people in our times were so obsessed with cutting carbs from their diet! What we know about protein today is a different story from previous times. Consuming an adequate amount of protein will help to promote more muscle mass, and it will help to preserve the muscle mass you currently have.

You might not care that much about muscle mass, but you definitely should. Muscle is more metabolically expensive than fat is. This means you'll burn more calories if you have more muscle on your frame.

Consuming enough protein will also help to promote satiety better than carbs or fat will, and it can have a greater effect from thermogenesis (25). Thermogenesis is the energy your body uses to digest and process the foods you eat. It's a cool little effect because you're burning calories just to process the foods you're eating.

With protein, you're essentially getting a bigger burn than from carbs or fat. Below are the estimated thermic effects for each macro (26):

Protein: 20-30%
Carbs: 5-10%
Fat: 0-3%

Essentially, this means if you ate 100 calories from protein, your body would burn off approximately 20-30 calories just to process that food. That is quite the difference if you consider that 100 calories from carbs would only burn 5-10 calories and fat 0-3 calories. Hopefully you can start to see the difference adequate protein intake makes when it comes to reaching your health and fitness goals.

If your diet consists primarily of simple carbs and unhealthy fats, you simply won't feel as satisfied, and you're missing out on some extra bonuses such as better thermogenesis. This is why consuming enough protein on a daily basis is a staple if you want to more easily get and stay in shape.

Consuming enough protein makes it harder for you to overconsume on things like simple carbs and unhealthy fats. Now let's discuss how much protein you should be consuming on a daily basis.

How Much Protein Should You Consume on a Regular Basis?

How much protein is the right amount for you so you're able to reap the benefits that I just mentioned? For the purposes of weight loss, I recommend consuming 40% of your total calories from protein. This may seem a bit high, but remember protein has a lot of benefits, and consuming enough protein is going to make everything else easier.

So then what about carbs and fat? I recommend an even split between those for fat loss purposes which brings each of those macros to 30% a piece. This is what your totals would look like:

40% of total calories from protein
30% of total calories from carbs
30% of total calories from fat

You can also discover how many calories from each macro you need to consume. Let's say you determine that you need to consume 1,850 calories per day in order to lose 1 pound per week. Here's how you can determine calories per macro:

1,850 x 0.4= 740 calories from protein
1,850 x 0.3= 555 calories from carbs
1,850 x 0.3= 555 calories from fat

You can then take things one step further and figure out the total number of grams. To figure this out, it's important to note that there are 4 calories per gram of protein, 4 calories per gram of carb, and 9 calories per gram of fat:

740/4= 185 grams of protein per day
555/4= 138.75 grams of carbs per day
555/9= 61.67 grams of fat per day

In a later chapter, I'm going to discuss more about tracking your macros and calories in a way that won't drive you crazy. For now, I just want to share with you some ideas of good food sources for each protein, carbs, and fat. This is by no means a comprehensive list. It's simply meant to help give you some ideas:

Protein:

- Chicken Breast
- Tuna
- Eggs
- Greek Yogurt
- Beef
- Cottage Cheese
- Turkey

Carbs:

- Brown Rice
- Sweet Potatoes
- Whole wheat pasta and bread
- Fruits
- Vegetables
- Oatmeal

Fats:

- Olive Oil
- Avocados
- Nuts
- Eggs

Chapter 6: Is Exercise Really All That Important?

When it comes to losing weight, what do you typically think of? Do you think of dieting? Do you think of running on the treadmill?

I think for most people, their mind goes to eating a salad and running on the treadmill in an effort to lose weight. Hopefully you've already been able to see that losing weight can be a lot more enjoyable than eating a bland salad all of the time. In this chapter, I'm here to do the same thing when it comes to exercise.

I want to show you that there's so much more to it than just walking or jogging on a cardio machine. There are a lot of benefits that you can gain from exercise when it's done in the correct manner.

You Can't Out Exercise a Bad Diet

Have you ever heard that you can't out exercise a bad diet? Maybe you have and maybe you haven't, but essentially, it means that it doesn't matter how much you exercise, if your diet is terrible then you will ultimately have no success in losing weight. Is there truth to this statement?

I definitely believe there is. Think of how easy it is to consume one small bag of potato chips that's roughly 150 calories. It's not hard to do at all!

Now think about what you would have to do in order to burn off those 150 calories you just ate. You'd have to walk approximately 1.5 miles in order to burn off those 150 calories! As you can clearly see, it's not practical to try and use exercise as a way to overcome bad eating habits.

This is why, ultimately, it's better to control your overall caloric intake via your nutrition. If you're allowed to eat 1,850 calories per day then it's better to figure out how to make those 150 calories from the potato chips a part of those original 1,850 calories. If you instead eat 2,000 calories because the potato chips were extra on top of your original 1,850, then it is unlikely you'll get around to burning those extra calories off from exercise.

Over time, this means you'll either lose weight at a slower rate, you won't lose weight at all, or you could even gain weight. With this being the case, you might be wondering what the benefit is to exercise? Why not just focus on diet and call it a day?

Yes, I would agree that nutrition makes up a larger percentage of your results when it comes to weight loss.

However, as you're about to see, there's more to exercise than simply burning some extra calories.

Why Does Exercise Matter Anyways?

If you want to lose weight, nutrition alone can get you to your goal. It would be foolish to use that as an excuse not to exercise though, if you're capable of doing so. There are so many benefits that come along with exercise that will essentially make it easier to get and stay in shape.

The Psychological Aspect of Working Out

To me, the most important reason for exercise is the mental benefit you get from it. Yes, exercise will release endorphins and make you feel good, but it's about so much more than just feeling good for a little bit after your workout. It's more so about the positive momentum you gain for the rest of the day.

How does the morning usually go for most people? They snooze and wake up at the last possible minute. Then they're rushed out the door without time to eat a proper breakfast.

It's also unlikely that they prepped a healthy breakfast the day prior or at the start of the week. This means that breakfast is either going to be skipped or the person is going to grab a quick fast food breakfast on the way to work.

If the person chose to skip breakfast, they're probably going to be hungry when break time rolls around and this could lead to some unhealthy snacking options at the vending machine.

The rushed person probably didn't consider anything for lunch either. So it's back to fast food when lunch rolls around. And what do you think is going to happen for dinner? Sure, it's possible that the person will cook for dinner, but it's also possible that after a long day of work, the person just wants to come home and relax.

The thought of having to think about what to eat, remember if all of the needed groceries are home or if a trip to the grocery store needs to be made, then cooking, and of course at some point the dishes are going to have to be cleaned. It's simply much easier to just get fast food again and not think about it. When you exercise, you can help to mitigate some of these issues purely because you don't want to ruin a good thing.

Imagine if you were eliminating miscellaneous spending for 30 days. If you've been able to stick to your goal for 14 days in a row, it's unlikely that you'll break it on the 15th day simply because you don't want to mess up your streak. Making one unnecessary purchase probably wouldn't be a big deal, but the streak you have going towards your ultimate goal is what would keep you on track.

Conversely, if you bought something unnecessary on day 3 of the challenge, then it would be much more likely that the floodgates would be open. You already spent money and broke the challenge so why not spend some more? The same type of thing occurs with eating when it comes to exercise.

Let's say this same person got up early instead of hitting the snooze button. They woke up and got a good workout in. Now they still have plenty of time to eat a good breakfast.

Let's assume this person didn't prep for lunch and didn't have time to make lunch before leaving for work. This person is going to have to go out for lunch, but it's more likely that healthier choices are going to be made. Maybe instead of going somewhere to get a burger and fries, they'll instead go to a salad bar or a healthy sandwich shop.

For dinner, even though it is going to require some effort, the person is more likely to cook because of the positive momentum brought forward from a simple action completed earlier in the day. Ultimately, I believe this is the best benefit of working out, and it doesn't matter what time of the day you workout.

You'll gain that positive momentum regardless of when you workout, and it can be used to help carry you through challenging moments such as when you're faced with eating unhealthy foods when you shouldn't.

Burning Some Extra Calories

Yes, as I explained earlier in this chapter, you can't out exercise a bad diet. Additionally, people usually don't burn as many calories as they think they are when exercising. For perspective, walking a mile will burn roughly 100 calories.

That's quite a bit of effort for a not so huge amount of calories. Even with these factors being the case, the fact that you can burn extra calories via exercise is pretty cool. Anytime you are able, you can exercise and burn some extra calories.

These calories likely won't be the difference between reaching your goal or missing it, however it still adds up. For instance, let's say you workout 4 times per week and burn an average of 200-250 calories per workout. On its own, that wouldn't seem like a lot, and I would agree.

However, that adds up to 800-1,000 additional calories burned over the week that you wouldn't have burned off otherwise. Over the course of the month, this would add up to about 3,200-4,000 extra calories burned, which is no small matter.

This means that you'll reach your end goal that much faster, or these calories can be viewed as a safety net. This way if your tracking is off slightly or if you consume more calories than you should on some days, you'll still stay on track to reach your goals.

Nutrient Partitioning

Nutrient partitioning is basically the process of how your body decides to use the calories you consume. Your body can use excess calories to go towards building muscle or they can go towards fat storage.

By exercising with resistance training, you can make your body more likely to have excess calories go towards helping repair your muscles. Compare this to someone who is very sedentary. Excess calories are most definitely going to be stored as fat.

The Lymphatic System

Your lymphatic system is part of your immune system and is responsible for helping regulate fluids in the body and dispose of waste from the body. Exercise helps to stimulate the lymphatic system and pump fluids throughout your body.

There are plenty more benefits to exercise than what I've talked about here.

Exercise is also good to help lower the risk for cardiovascular disease (27), but the main point is that you're better off with exercise than without it, regardless of what your goals are.

Exercise and Metabolic Adaptation

You've already learned about how metabolic adaptation works in regards to your diet, but does it apply to the way you exercise as well? As it turns out, it definitely does! You can use exercise to train your metabolism to burn more or less calories depending on how you exercise.

For instance, let's say the only kind of exercising you do is long distance cardio. You're essentially training your metabolism to burn less calories because it needs to be more efficient. One way your body will do this is by burning muscle.

With long distance type of cardio, you're signaling to your body that you don't need the muscle to lift heavy things so it can "get rid" of it to make the metabolism more efficient (aka slow down) and instead focus more on improving endurance. On the other hand, when you perform resistance training, you're telling your body that muscle is needed to lift heavy things.

It will adapt and build more muscle. More muscle means more calories burned since it is metabolically expensive to maintain muscle.

You're training your metabolism to become inefficient, which is what we want for the goal of fat loss.

If the goal was purely survival then having a very efficient metabolism that burns less calories would be great because we could eat less to survive. That's not the problem in modern times though. Here are a couple of examples to help illustrate this point.

Imagine if you did 30 jump squats in a row. You might be pretty gassed afterwards. Now, let's say you continued to do 30 jump squats once a day for 3 months.

As time goes on, you would get less fatigued from this bout of exercise because your body is adapting to it. You would also burn less calories by the end of the third month compared to when you first started. This isn't a bad thing, your body is doing what it does best, adapting!

Now compare that to if you did one max effort jump per day. Your body is focused on being as explosive as possible and gaining more explosiveness not being more efficient with the number of calories burned. You can also think of this in terms of cars.

Imagine a drag race that lasts only 10 seconds. These cars go extremely fast but they burn a ton of fuel in the process.

This isn't a problem because the goal isn't fuel efficiency; it's to go as fast as possible for a short distance.

However, if you were going on a road trip, you would not want to use a vehicle that's used for a drag race. You'd rather use a fuel efficient car that gets great miles per gallon. However, cars that get good gas mileage aren't exactly explosive like other cars such as sports cars, for example.

They're less fuel efficient and burn through more gas. Think of your metabolism like a car. The more gas a car burns through is like your metabolism burning through more calories.

This will give you more leeway to eat more and still create a caloric deficit. Finally, you can also think of this in terms of how certain people's bodies look. Look at the difference in how a typical marathon runner looks compared to a sprinter.

A marathon runner is going to have very little muscle mass and is trained for endurance. A sprinter, on the other hand, is going to have quite a bit more muscle and is training for explosiveness. On average, a sprinter's metabolism is going to be higher than a marathon runner's metabolism.

This isn't to say that cardio has no place as part of a proper exercise regime.

Rather, you have to be strategic with how you're doing your cardio to ensure you get the most out of it without it hindering your metabolism. First things first though, let's go more in depth on resistance training...

The Importance of Resistance Training

I've already touched on some of the benefits that exercise is going to provide you. Cardio and strength training have their mutual and exclusive benefits. However, I want to go more in depth on the importance of lifting weights in regards to what it can provide you.

On the surface, you might not be that interested in resistance training. You might think that it's not for you or that it's something for meatheads at the gym. It definitely can be, but it doesn't have to be that way.

For starters, the best benefit to lifting weights is that it allows your body to build more muscle. As you've already learned, our bodies are adaptation machines. If you give your body a stimulus to grow bigger and stronger, it will absolutely do so.

So in the case of weight lifting, you're breaking down your muscles. Your body then says, "wow I don't want to undergo a stress like this ever again." So your body will then work to repair itself.

It will regrow the muscle back bigger and stronger so that it won't be under that same level of stress again. This is why it's actually during the recovery process that your body grows back bigger and stronger. When you workout, you break down your muscles.

Then you recover and repair your body to grow back bigger and stronger. Again, why does that matter? Your goal might not be to become a competitive bodybuilder, so why should you care?

It all comes down to what the muscle can do for you. Namely, a higher metabolism makes it easier for you to lose fat and keep it off. If you had the choice between eating more calories or less calories in order to lose weight, what would you choose?

You would obviously choose eating more calories, and lifting weights gives you the ability to be able to do just that! Not only that, but it looks good. Having the right amount of muscle in the right places does look nice.

You don't need to be a competitive bodybuilder, but you might want to strive to improve the look of your body. Many women, for instance, want to tone their bodies. I think this is a great goal, but the truth is that you can't technically "tone" your body. All you can do is the following:

-Gain fat

-Burn fat
-Gain muscle
-Lose muscle

Therefore, toning is simply a combination of burning fat and gaining a slight amount of muscle. For most people, if all they did was just lose weight, they still might not be satisfied with how they look. Adding some muscle can help with that.

We can also use resistance training to help correct imbalances that present themselves in the body. If left untreated, these imbalances can eventually manifest in the form of various issues such as lower back pain or knee pain among many other things.

Sample Beginner Resistance Training Workout

-Chest Press Machine: 3 sets, 10 reps, 45 seconds rest between sets
-Leg Press Machine: 3 sets, 12 reps, 30 seconds rest between sets
-Seated Row Machine: 3 sets, 10 reps, 45 seconds rest between sets
-Shoulder Press Machine: 3 sets, 12 reps, 30 seconds rest between sets
-Ab Crunch Machine: 3 sets, 15 reps, 30 seconds rest between sets

Complete this workout three times per week with at least one day of rest in between workouts.

Note: Reps are the number of times you perform the exercise. A set is one complete round of repetitions. For example, on the chest press machine you would lift the weight 10 times to complete your first set. Then you would rest for 45 seconds and start the second set. You would then repeat this process one more time to complete the third set and then move onto the next exercise.

Why Does This Workout Consist of Nothing But Machines?

You might be wondering why this workout consists of nothing but machines. It's first important to understand the difference between machines and free weights. Typically, most commercial gyms will be divided and have a machine section and a free weight section.

Free weight exercises are exercises that are performed using equipment such as dumbbells, barbells, kettlebells, or even your own bodyweight. It's pretty self-explanatory what a machine is. Popular gym machines you've probably seen before are things such as a leg extension, hamstring curl, or chest press machine.

So what's the difference, and why does it matter? With a machine, you're going to be locked into place. All you have to do is move in a certain way to complete the exercise.

There's very little room for error when it comes to correctly performing an exercise via a machine. For instance, on the chest press machine, you simply grab the handles and press them forward until your arms are fully extended. It's very hard to mess up the exercise.

This is why I think that machines are great for beginners who may be brand new to the gym and resistance training. Not only that, but machines are less intimidating. Usually, the more experienced weight lifters will be in the free weight section, and it can be intimidating for some people who are brand new to venture into that area at the start.

Not only is the machine section less scary, but it's far less likely that you'll feel foolish or worry that you're not performing an exercise correctly in front of everyone else at the gym. Sadly, when it comes to the benefits that machines can provide to you, this is about as far as they go.

This isn't to say that these benefits are negligible because that's far from the truth, but most fitness experts would agree that free weights are superior to machines.

This is why you'll usually see the more experienced lifters spend most of their time in the gym at the free weight section as opposed to the machine section. So what is it that makes free weights so much better?

The main thing it boils down to is stabilizer muscles. For instance, let's compare a seated shoulder press machine to a seated shoulder press performed with dumbbells. In the case of the machine, the bars can't move out to the side, forwards or backwards.

They're locked into place so you only have to focus on pressing them upwards. In the case of the dumbbells, you must stabilize them throughout the movement to prevent them from going to the side, forwards or backwards. If you're lifting really light weights that don't challenge you, stabilizing the weight won't be hard at all.

However, as you start to lift some heavier weights that are challenging for your current fitness level, you will definitely start to notice the difference between a free weight version of an exercise compared to a machine version. In the long run, this will translate to more calories burned from exercise and more strength where it's needed.

For athletes, this means you could be less likely to sustain an injury, and the average person is less likely to develop imbalances or weaknesses that could cause problems down the road. Additionally, free weights also allow you to move the weight in a way that's more comfortable for your particular body.

For instance, when I perform the flat dumbbell bench press exercise, I like to keep my elbows tucked at a 45 degree angle as opposed to 90 degrees. In the case of a machine, you're not able to change how the bar or handles are positioned. Your body has to conform to the machine instead of making the weights conform to how you want to lift them.

Free weights aren't without their downsides. The biggest downside to free weights is the potential to cause injury. The main reason the potential is so high is because there are more technicalities to performing free weight exercises.

You must have good technique when lifting with free weights or else you'll expose yourself to possibly sustaining an injury. Injury when exercising is the last thing you want. It will keep you out of the gym and that means you're not getting any of the benefits from exercise that I mentioned earlier.

It's certainly enough to knock people off track, and it can be hard to get that momentum back. Most injuries in the gym occur because people get too ambitious with how much weight they're lifting. Once you start lifting a weight that is too heavy for you, your form is likely to be compensated in order for you to be able to complete the lift.

Keep in mind, your body doesn't know what good form is. All it knows is that it's dealing with a heavy weight that needs to be moved from point A to point B. So if there's a way to shorten that distance, your body is going to take that path even if it puts other muscles in jeopardy.

If your body needs to get other muscles involved that shouldn't have anything to do with a certain exercise, it will do so as well. Take a standard barbell curl, for instance. Sometimes you'll see people cheat the weight up by swinging their elbows forward and leaning back to get momentum to help get the weight up.

The problem with this is now you're involving your shoulders when this is supposed to be a bicep exercise. Additionally, the excessive leaning backwards is putting the lower back at risk for injury. Try cheating on a bicep concentration curl machine, and you'll notice it's very hard to do so!

I'm not trying to scare you away from free weights, you just need to be mindful that technique is of the utmost importance when it comes to free weights. If proper lifting form is used, you'll be able to reap the benefits of free weights for a long time to come. So with all of that being said, if you're brand new to the gym, it's okay to start out with machines to dip your feet in the water and get used to things.

That's why I recommend that you use the above workout as a good way to get started. Eventually though, you will want to transition into a workout that is mostly centered around free weights. You can, of course, also use machines to help supplement your workout such as fully exhausting a muscle group at the end of your workout.

The biggest thing that keeps people stuck on the treadmill or in the machine section at the gym is intimidation. So let's cover how you can overcome that fear.

Over to Overcome the Fear of Intimidation at the Gym

Feeling scared or intimidated at the gym is a totally normal feeling. It's a brand new environment, and you don't want to look foolish. I went through the same thing.

My first semester of college, I actually worked out entirely in my tiny dorm room with resistance bands simply because I was afraid of navigating the rec center and looking silly. Keep in mind, I was in athletics all throughout high school, and my major was in Kinesiology so I should've been fearless!

So what can you do if you're worried about the same thing happening to you, or maybe it's something that has held you back in the past? Well first of all, the gym you go to matters. Some gyms cater more to beginners.

Other gyms focus on a specific group of people. A lot of times, these specific gyms will naturally have more experienced people go to them simply by the nature of the gym. It's not that any gym is trying to exclude a certain group of people, but the strengths of certain gyms cater to a more experienced crowd.

In your case, if you're on the beginner side of things, make sure you go to a gym that is beginner friendly. There will still be people who look intimidating, but they will be far less than at other gyms. So make sure you do a thorough investigation of gyms in your area to decide which one is best for you.

Take a tour during the busiest time such as 5-7 PM to see what different types of fitness levels are there. This should give you a good idea and allow you to make an informed decision. Once you've picked out your gym, the next thing I recommend you do is go during a time when the gym isn't as crowded.

If your schedule allows you to workout sometime during the day when most people are at work, that would be ideal. However, that's not going to be the case for a lot of people. The gym will be less crowded in the morning before work compared to the evening once work is over.

Once you're at the gym, stick to the machine section. This will help get you in the habit of going to the gym and being more comfortable simply being in a gym environment. Over time, you should start to feel comfortable with the layout of the gym, how gym etiquette works, and simply feel a sense of belonging and that this is a part of who you are and what you do.

Once you start to gain that feeling, it's time to venture over to the free weight section. There are a couple of ways to go about doing this. If you have a friend you could bring with you who is experienced, that's a potential option.

This person can not only help guide you in regards to technique but also just help you feel more comfortable.

If you don't have a friend in this sense then start off small. Go during a time when the gym isn't crowded.

All you need to do is perform 1-2 free weight exercises. Simply do what you're comfortable with. If you want to complete an exercise that involves a bench, that is great.

If not, you can simply grab a pair of dumbbells and perform standing dumbbell curls in an open area in the free weight section. Over time, you will start to get more comfortable in that part of the gym. Start small and build your way up. Don't feel as if you have to go from nothing but machines to nothing but free weights. Just dip your toes in the water, and take things one step at a time. Finally, the last thing I want to remind you of is that no one really cares.

Everyone is focused on what they're doing at the gym. No one is hyper focused on what you're doing at the gym. To prove my point, when you go to the gym, how closely are you paying attention to what everyone else is doing?

How much are you thinking about what everyone else is doing? I'm willing to bet that you're more focused on what you need to be doing at the gym as opposed to thinking about what others are doing. The same goes for other people at the gym!

Even if you do mess up, don't worry about it. It's about going out there and giving your best effort that you can be proud of. If someone else laughs at you or judges you, that's on them and their character. Stay focused on yourself at the gym and do what you can to improve upon your current fitness level. That's what matters!

Free Weight Beginner Workout at the Gym

Once you've become more accustomed to the gym and are ready to incorporate free weights as part of your regular routine, the following is a great beginner weight workout you can follow:

-Goblet Squat: 3 sets, 10 reps, 60 seconds rest between sets
-Incline Dumbbell Chest Press: 3 sets, 10 reps, 60 seconds rest between sets
-Lat Pulldown: 3 sets, 12 reps, 45 seconds rest between sets
-Seated Dumbbell Military Press: 3 sets, 10 reps, 60 seconds rest between sets
-Incline Dumbbell Curls: 3 sets, 12 reps, 45 seconds rest between sets
-Dumbbell Skull Crushers: 3 sets, 12 reps, 45 seconds rest between sets
-Wood Chops: 3 sets, 10 reps per side, 30 seconds rest between sets

Complete this workout 3 times per week, taking at least one day of rest in between each workout.

Free Weight Intermediate Workout at the Gym

Day 1: Chest, Shoulders, Triceps

-Stability Ball Chest Press: 3 sets, 8 reps, 60 seconds rest between sets
-One Arm Standing Kettlebell Press: 3 sets, 8 reps per arm, 60 seconds rest between sets
-Ez Bar Skull Crushers: 3 sets, 10 reps, 45 seconds rest between sets
-Cable Chest Fly High Finish: 3 sets, 12 reps, 30 seconds rest between sets
-Standing Dumbbell Lateral Raises: 3 sets, 12 reps, 30 seconds rest between sets
-Overhead Cable Extension: 3 sets, 15 reps, 30 seconds rest between sets
-Ab Wheel Rollouts: 3 sets, as many rollouts as possible, 45 seconds rest between sets

Day 2: Back, Biceps, Legs

-Bulgarian Split Squats: 3 sets, 8 reps per leg, 45 seconds rest between sets
-Pull-Ups (bodyweight or weighted): 3 sets, 8 reps, 60 seconds rest between sets
-Ez Bar Curls: 3 sets, 8 reps, 60 seconds rest between sets
-Stability Ball Hamstring Curls: 3 sets, 12 reps Super Set with Wall Sits 3 sets Max Hold, 60 seconds rest between sets

-Seated Cable Rows: 3 sets, 10 reps, 45 seconds rest between sets
-Cross Body Hammer Curls: 3 sets, 10 reps per arm, 45 seconds rest per set
-Hanging Knee Ups: 3 sets, 10 reps, 60 seconds rest between sets

Complete each workout two times per week alternating between day 1 and day 2. Here are a couple of ways you can set your workout schedule:

Monday: Chest, Shoulders, Triceps
Tuesday: Back, Biceps, Legs
Wednesday: Rest Day
Thursday: Chest, Shoulders, Triceps
Friday: Back, Biceps, Legs
Saturday: Rest Day
Sunday: Rest Day

Or

Monday: Chest, Shoulders, Triceps
Tuesday: Back, Biceps, Legs
Wednesday: Rest Day
Thursday: Chest, Shoulders, Triceps
Friday: Rest Day
Saturday: Back, Biceps, Legs
Sunday: Rest Day

If you're unsure if you should start with the beginner workout or intermediate, I would recommend starting with the beginner workout unless you have at least one year of workout experience under your belt.

Functional Exercises

One thing you may have noticed is that the intermediate workout contains more exercises done on stability balls or single leg exercises. Some people might refer to these types of exercises as functional exercises. What's meant by this is that there's more carryover to day-to-day life or for sports athletes when compared to other exercises.

It also allows you to train your body in a way that can help combat day-to-day tendencies. For example, a lot of people in the modern day work desk jobs and sit a lot throughout the day. Excessive sitting can cause tight hip flexors, weak abs, and weak glutes.

To help combat this, you can utilize exercises that get the glutes more involved. For instance, when working on your chest, you could perform a regular flat dumbbell bench press. This exercise wouldn't involve the glutes at all.

It's not a bad exercise by any means; it simply isn't as practical given most people sit a lot, which causes their glutes to be inactive.

You could also perform the same exercise on a stability ball and use your glutes to stabilize your body and help maintain a 90 degree angle at your knees. Now you're being more efficient with your time and getting the most out of every exercise that you do.

Another example is performing single arm or single leg exercises. Performing an exercise on both sides of the body at the same time is referred to as a bilateral exercise. Performing an exercise one side at a time is a unilateral exercise.

Unilateral exercises require more stability. The opposite side from the side that's working must work hard to stabilize your body to prevent it from tilting over. However, one downside of unilateral exercises compared to bilateral exercises is that you won't be able to lift as much weight.

As with most things, there is a give and take. For the average person though, incorporating more exercises that involve the core and glutes is going to be a good thing.

What if You Need to Workout From Home?

I understand that it may not be practical for everyone to be able to go to a commercial gym and workout.

There's definitely a lot more you can do at a gym, however don't be fooled into thinking that working out from home is a waste of time because it certainly isn't. The following is an effective bodyweight workout you can do from the comfort of your own home:

-Bodyweight Squats: 3 sets, 20 reps, 20 seconds rest between sets
-Pushups: 3 sets, 20 reps, 20 seconds rest between sets
-Mountain Climbers: 3 sets, 30 seconds, 20 seconds rest between sets
-Glute Bridges: 3 sets, 10 reps, 30 seconds rest between sets
-High Knees: 3 sets, 30 seconds, 20 seconds rest between sets
-Close Grip Push-ups: 3 sets, 15 reps, 30 seconds rest between sets
-Scissor Jacks: 3 sets, 20 reps, 20 seconds rest between sets
-Plank: 3 sets, max hold, 30 seconds rest between sets

The thing I love about bodyweight workouts is that you can do them just about anywhere. You don't have to be bound to a specific location like a gym or have access to certain equipment. The downside is that it can be more difficult to make bodyweight workouts a challenge when compared to gym workouts.

In the case of this bodyweight workout, you can easily adapt things to meet your current fitness level. You can do this by lowering the number of reps completed for each exercise or increasing rest time, as needed, to make things easier. If you need more of a challenge, you can increase reps, decrease rest time, and/or superset exercises.

A superset is where you complete two exercises back to back without any rest until the second exercise is completed. In this workout, for instance, you could superset bodyweight squats with push-ups to make things more of a challenge.

Dumbbell Only Home Workout

The following is a workout you can do from home with only a pair of dumbbells:

Floor Press: 3 sets, 15 reps, 30 seconds rest between sets
Dumbbell Squat: 3 sets, 15 reps, 45 seconds rest between sets
Standing Dumbbell Shoulder Press: 3 sets, 10 reps, 30 seconds rest between sets
Renegade Row: 3 sets, 6 reps per side, 45 seconds rest between sets
Skull Crushers on floor: 3 sets, 15 reps, 30 seconds rest between sets
Standing Dumbbell Curls: 3 sets, 10 reps, 30 seconds rest between sets

Side plank: 3 sets, max hold each side, 30 seconds rest between sets

If you only have one pair of dumbbells, you may need to increase the amount of reps or decrease rest time on certain exercises to make them more challenging. For instance, let's say you own one 20-pound pair of dumbbells. You'll be able to lift more weight on the floor press exercise, which is essentially a bench press performed on the floor, than you would be able to lift for the dumbbell curls.

Therefore, you'll need to make those 20-pound dumbbells more of a challenge, which you can do by shortening rest periods or increasing reps. If you currently don't have any home gym equipment and are interested in where to start, I'd say the best place is with an adjustable pair of dumbbells.

This will save space and give you lots of versatility when it comes to exercises. From there, I'd get an adjustable bench to give you access to even more exercises. Those are the two basics I would start with. Then if space allows for it, you could get a barbell with weight plates and then a squat rack.

How to Warm-Up Before Lifting Weights

When you're lifting weights, warming up is critical. By skipping a warm-up, you're putting yourself at a higher risk to sustain an injury. Think about any athlete.

Do they just jump right into the game? No, of course not! You'll see them out on the field or court warming up well before the actual game starts.

The same premise needs to be applied to lifting weights. If you can bench press 225 pounds, it doesn't make sense to jump straight into that. Instead, you need to work your way up to that to help prevent injuries from occurring. The following is a good general warm-up you can do to help get blood flowing throughout your body:

Light jog on treadmill or cardio machine of choice for 5 minutes (jump rope or air jump rope if cardio machine is unavailable or you're unable to jog outside)
Big Circle Forward Arm Swings for 20 seconds
Small Circle Forward Arm Swings for 20 seconds
Big Circle Backwards Arm Swings for 20 seconds
Small Circle Backwards Arm Swings for 20 seconds
Jumping Jacks for 20 reps
Push-Ups for 15 reps
Bodyweight Squats for 15 reps

Once you complete this, you'll also want to make sure that you do some warm-up sets for your big compound lifts such as your weighted squats or the bench press. For instance, let's say on the dumbbell squat exercise you normally use 50-pound dumbbells in each hand. It doesn't make sense to jump straight into using the 50-pound dumbbells for your 3 main working sets.
Instead, do 2 warm-up sets to get ready for your working sets. So in this case, you might use 25-pound dumbbells and perform 10 reps. After resting for one minute, you could then use 40-pound dumbbells for 5 reps. Take a final rest for 1-2 minutes, and now you should be ready to go for your first main set.

Should You Completely Avoid Cardio?

As I mentioned earlier, too much cardio can lead to your metabolism slowing down. It's better to focus on being explosive. So does this mean you should avoid cardio all together?

The answer to this is no, definitely not! You just have to be smart about the way you go about it. Most people think of cardio as something that is slow, long, and boring and typically done on a treadmill.

However, if you want to keep your metabolism humming along then you'll want to avoid this. Instead, focus on training more so along the lines of how a sprinter would. A sprinter doesn't train by running at the same pace for a long period of time; rather, a sprinter goes all out, takes a rest, and then does it again.

This allows for each run to be at max effort. For the average person, a good way to mimic this style of training is by performing high intensity interval training. The name is pretty self-explanatory. You train at high intensities, but you do so at intervals.

For instance, you might run at 8 miles per hour for one minute and then walk at a pace of 3.5 miles per hour for 90 seconds, and repeat that for 7 rounds. The cool thing about this workout is that you can adjust it to fit your needs. Let's say running at 8 miles per hour for one minute is too challenging for you.

You can lower the speed and/or duration as needed. So you might run at a pace of 6.5 mph for 45 seconds instead of 8 miles per hour for one minute straight. You can also increase or decrease the lower intensity cardio as well.

Instead of walking for 90 seconds, you could walk for 60 seconds or walk for 2 minutes. Adjust things to where you're currently at, and strive to improve things as you go.

If you start out doing 6.5 miles per hour for 45 seconds followed by a 2 minute walk at 3 miles per hour for 7 rounds, then strive to cut the walk interval down to 90 seconds or to increase your speed up to 7 miles per hour.

There are a lot of different variables that you can play around with. The other cool thing about this type of cardio workout is that you can do it on basically any type of cardio machine or even outside where space allows. This can be done on an elliptical, rower, treadmill, track, field, or anywhere else.

This is a great type of workout to do if you don't have access to any type of cardio equipment. Strive to perform this high intensity interval training workout at least 2-3 times per week in addition to your resistance training workout.

How to Implement Weight Training with Cardio

So ideally, you should be performing resistance training at least 3 times per week, and you should also implement high intensity interval training 2-3 times per week as well to help keep the metabolism high and create some extra calorie burning. The question is how do you fit it all in? Well, that really depends on you and what works best for your schedule.

If it works out better for you to do your resistance training on separate days from your cardio then do that. So you might lift weights on Mondays, Wednesdays, and Fridays and then perform high intensity interval training on Tuesdays and Thursdays. You could also choose to perform both on the same day.

In this case, that would be something along the lines of performing your weight workout first and then immediately following it with your cardio workout on Mondays, Wednesdays, and Fridays. If you choose this option, make sure that you always perform your weight training first. You'll notice that you'll be able to lift heavier weights this way.

If you complete your cardio first, you'll be fatigued and your weight training workout will suffer. Sure, you might not be able to run quite as fast after an intense weight workout, but it will be less affected than the weight workout will be by the cardio.

Chapter 7: Tying It All Together

In this last chapter, I want to put together the final pieces to help you complete the puzzle that is the metabolic confusion diet. The first step to be able to do this all comes down to the way you prepare.

Preparation Above All Else

By this point in the book, you now have knowledge that most people will sadly never know, and it comes down to execution, at this point. We can have the best of intentions, but sometimes our intentions can get pushed to the side when life happens. Unexpected things happen at work and we end up staying late.

Now there's less time to cook. We might plan on meal prepping on Sunday, but then we get carried away watching football only to wonder where the day went. We have to be prepared for things like this to happen and plan in advance.

We have to make preparation as easy as possible or else we will still fail. For instance, when it comes to grocery shopping, getting your groceries delivered to your door is a great option, if possible. Even if you're unable to do that, a lot of grocery stores now days offer curbside pickup.

Either one of these two options are highly recommended for a few reasons. The first is that the grocery store can seem daunting at times. This can sometimes cause us to delay going, which means we won't be prepared and make us more likely to eat fast food.

Secondly, grocery delivery or curbside pickup allows you to stay focused. You'll be ordering your groceries online, which means you'll be far less likely to suddenly see something at the store and buy it on impulse. Ordering your groceries ahead of time can save time that could then be used to help prep your meals.

As far as meal prepping is concerned, you should definitely do it. Trying to meal prep the day of or day before can be a little risky because you never know what can pop up. Something unexpected is bound to occur sooner or later, and it can throw your schedule out of whack.

If you're then unable to meal prep, you're now set up for failure. My advice would be to meal prep either on Sunday or split it up between Sunday and Wednesday.

Counting Calories and Macros

In this book, I've talked about how many calories you should eat and ideal macro ratios.

It's cool and all to know how many calories you should be eating on a daily basis, but it's a whole different battle to know how many calories you're actually eating. The only way to know how many calories you're eating is to track them.

As the old phase goes, "what gets measured gets managed," and this is so true. This is how you'll know that you're on the right track. If you simply wing it, you'll be left wondering why the weight on the scale isn't going down.

Tracking calories is very important for when you take your diet break. You want to ensure you're eating enough calories on these days to help prevent metabolic slowdown. The last thing you want is to accidentally undereat during your diet break.

Yes, it will be tedious at first, but just know that it will get better as time goes on. You'll eventually start to develop an eye for how many calories certain foods contain. It will also be easy to track meals that you regularly eat. Be patient with yourself. Understand that you will never be perfect with it, and that's okay. Here are some tips to help you out:

Don't Be Spot On

You don't need to be spot on when it comes to your tracking. That would make any normal person go bonkers. Instead, aim to be within 5-10% of the actual caloric amount.

For instance, if a food item actually contains 200 calories, your goal is to track between 180-220 calories.

Overestimate When You're Not Sure

You're trying to lose weight, and we have a tendency to underestimate the amount of calories we eat by quite a bit as it turns out (28). Therefore, if you want to be successful, do the opposite of what most people do and overestimate.

If you think something contains 300 calories but you're not quite sure, add 10% just to be on the safe side. This way you'll still stay on track to reach your goals. Worst case scenario, if you did overestimate, you'll at least reach your end goal a little bit sooner.

Focus Only on Calories and Protein If You Have To

If the thought of tracking your calories and macros seems too overwhelming to you, just focus on your overall caloric intake and the amount of protein you're consuming. You can eventually work your way into tracking carbs and fat, but it's not critical that you do so right off the bat. It's better to not be overwhelmed and do what is simpler.

By tracking your overall calories, you can ensure that you're in a deficit. Tracking your protein will help to prevent muscle loss, help with satiety, and help keep your metabolism high. That's why it's more important to track overall calories and protein than carbs and fat.

Use an App

There are plenty of calorie and macro tracking apps out there, and a lot of them have similar features. Try a few different ones out to see what you like best. Using apps with a bar code scanner will make tracking super simple.

Once you scan the barcode, all of the nutritional information will pop up right in the app. You'll also have the ability to save meals. So if you eat something more than once, all of the information will be saved allowing for you to do a quick add the next time you eat that meal.

Some apps even have a feature that allows you to take a picture of your meal, and it will calculate the calories and macros for that meal automatically. That will definitely make your life easier when it comes to tracking.

Sample Day of Eating

The following is a sample way to give you an example of what a typical day of eating might look like:

Weekday:

Breakfast: Protein Shake consisting of two scoops of whey protein, 0.5 cup of oatmeal, 1.5 cups of oat milk, 1 frozen banana, 0.5 cup of greek yogurt, and a handful of spinach (don't worry you won't taste it)

Lunch: Grilled Chicken Salad

Dinner: Whole Wheat Spaghetti with a side of brussel sprouts

Weekend:

Breakfast: Oatmeal with honey and whey protein

Lunch: Sandwich consisting of whole wheat bread, one slice of cheese, mustard, pickles, and over the deli honey ham with a small bag of potato chips

Dinner: Eat a meal at your favorite restaurant

Conclusion

Well, that's it! Congratulations on making it to the end of this book. You now hold the keys to unlocking the most fit version of yourself, and be proud of that because most people will never have that opportunity.

They will sadly spin their wheels losing weight only to gain it back and never realize the trap their own bodies have put them in. You, on the other hand, are different. You now know how to break free from that cycle, and you can do so by following these core principles discussed throughout the book:

-Take a break from dieting every so often (every 3-4 weeks is a good spot for most people)
-Don't try to lose weight too quickly (0.5-2 pounds per week is ideal for most people)
-Consume enough protein per day
-Incorporate resistance training as part of your exercise regime

Write these four key points down, and post them on your desk, fridge, or wherever else you have to! I want you to constantly be reminded of these points and never lose sight of them. It might get tempting at times to want to lose weight at a faster pace or to skip your diet break, but that would be a big mistake!

Stay patient, stick to the process, and eventually before you know it, you'll be amazed at how far you've come. There's not much left to say other than go out there and crush it!

References:

1. https://www.cdc.gov/obesity/data/adult.html
2. https://study.com/academy/lesson/how-seligmans-learned-helplessness-theory-applies-to-human-depression-and-stress.html
3. https://en.wikipedia.org/wiki/Four-minute_mile
4. https://earthobservatory.nasa.gov/features/OrbitsHistory#:~:text=In%201543%2C%20Nicolaus%20Copernicus%20detailed,century%20to%20become%20widely%20accepted.
5. https://www.biggerpockets.com/blog/2015-11-06-set-goals-for-2016
6. https://www.ncbi.nlm.nih.gov/pmc/articles/PMC4377487/#:~:text=The%20regulation%20and%20metabolism%20of,with%20sleep%20and%20circadian%20rhythmicity
7. https://pubmed.ncbi.nlm.nih.gov/18564298/
8. https://pubmed.ncbi.nlm.nih.gov/20020365/#:~:text=Growth%20hormone%20is%20primarily%20known,metabolic%20functions%20throughout%20adult%20life.
9. https://pubmed.ncbi.nlm.nih.gov/8627466/#:~:text=Sleep%2Drelated%20secretion%20of%20GH,decrease%20wakefulness%20and%20increase%20SWS.

10. https://www.cdc.gov/sleep/about_sleep/how_much_sleep.html
11. https://www.cdc.gov/media/releases/2016/p0215-enough-sleep.html
12. https://news.gallup.com/poll/166553/less-recommended-amount-sleep.aspx#:~:text=PRINCETON%2C%20NJ%20%2D%2D%20Fifty%2Dnine,get%20less%20than%20seven%20hours.
13. https://pubmed.ncbi.nlm.nih.gov/29784810/
14. https://pubmed.ncbi.nlm.nih.gov/30827911/
15. https://onlinelibrary.wiley.com/doi/full/10.1111/jsr.12712
16. https://pubmed.ncbi.nlm.nih.gov/21075238/
17. https://pubmed.ncbi.nlm.nih.gov/13594881/
18. https://www.ncbi.nlm.nih.gov/pmc/articles/PMC5747444/
19. https://pubmed.ncbi.nlm.nih.gov/22209501/
20. https://pubmed.ncbi.nlm.nih.gov/10349584/
21. https://www.ncbi.nlm.nih.gov/pmc/articles/PMC3551118/
22. https://pubmed.ncbi.nlm.nih.gov/2761578/
23. https://pubmed.ncbi.nlm.nih.gov/23729611/
24. Https://www.ket.org/program/in-defense-of-food/dr-kellogg-and-the-crusade-against-protein/

25. https://pubmed.ncbi.nlm.nih.gov/1846929287/
26. https://nutritionandmetabolism.biomedcentral.com/articles/10.1186/1743-7075-1-5#citeas
27. https://pubmed.ncbi.nlm.nih.gov/30324108/
28. https://pubmed.ncbi.nlm.nih.gov/1454084/

Printed in Great Britain
by Amazon

20149396R00088